5TH EDITION

FIRST AID
MANUAL

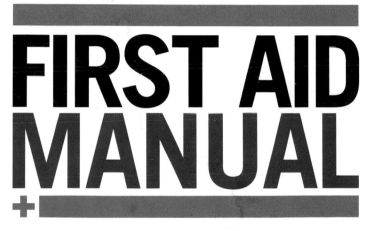

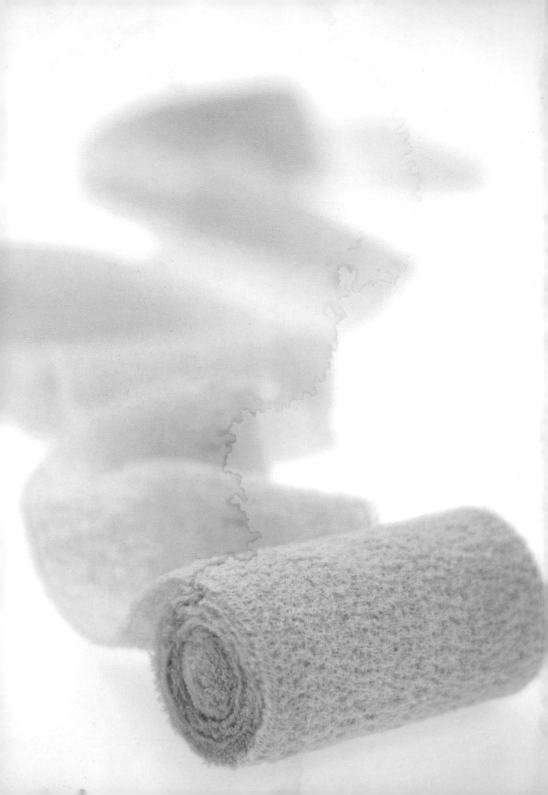

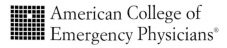
American College of
Emergency Physicians®

ADVANCING EMERGENCY CARE

5TH EDITION

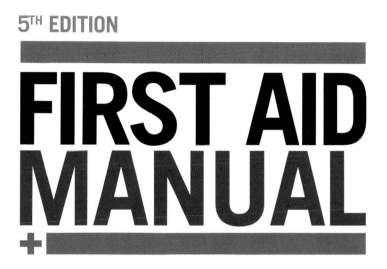

FIRST AID MANUAL

Medical Editor-in-Chief **Gina M. Piazza, DO, FACEP**

LONDON, NEW YORK, MUNICH, MELBOURNE, DELHI

DORLING KINDERSLEY

Consultant editor Jemima Dunne	**Senior art editor** Spencer Holbrook
Senior editor Janet Mohun	**Jacket designer** Duncan Turner
Jacket editor Maud Whatley	**Producer** Vivienne Yong
US senior editor Margaret Parrish	**Photography** Gerard Brown, Vanessa Davies, Ruth Jenkinson
US editor Jill Hamilton	
Pre-production producer Francesca Wardell	**Jacket design development manager** Sophia MTT
Managing editor Angeles Gavira Guerrero	**Managing art editor** Michelle Baxter
Publisher Sarah Larter	**Art director** Philip Ormerod
Associate publishing director Liz Wheeler	**Publishing director** Jonathan Metcalf

AMERICAN COLLEGE OF EMERGENCY PHYSICIANS

Medical Editor-in-Chief Gina M. Piazza, DO, FACEP	**Associate Executive Director, Membership and Education Division** Robert Heard, MBA, CAE
	Director, Educational Products Marta Foster

Text revised in line with the latest guidelines from the Resuscitation Council (US).

Fifth edition first published in the United States in 2014 by
DK Publishing, 4th floor, 345 Hudson Street, New York, NY 10014

14 15 16 17 18 10 9 8 7 6 5 4 3 2 1
001–192570–September/2014

DK books are available at special discounts when purchased in bulk for sales promotions, premiums, fund-raising, or educational use. For details, contact: DK Publishing Special Markets, 345 Hudson Street, New York, New York 10014 or SpecialSales@dk.com.

Printed and bound in China by Leo

Discover more at
www.dk.com

FOREWORD

THE AMERICAN COLLEGE OF EMERGENCY PHYSICIANS (ACEP)

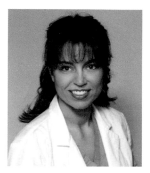

GINA M. PIAZZA, DO, FACEP
MEDICAL EDITOR-IN-CHIEF

The goal of the American College of Emergency Physicians (ACEP) is to support high-quality emergency care throughout our country. More than 130 million persons come to hospital emergency departments every year, seeking care for everything from mild illnesses and injuries to life-threatening conditions. Emergency care is provided in a continuum that starts with the bystander who first recognizes a problem and begins treatment, through the care rendered by emergency medical services (EMS) personnel, to the care provided in hospital emergency departments nationwide.

Either directly or indirectly, every citizen is affected by injury or illness at some point. It is important for all of us to be able to recognize emergency medical events and to possess the basic knowledge and skills necessary to summon appropriate help and to provide basic care until that help arrives. The goal of this manual is to instruct you in these basic skills and to provide you with the knowledge you need to make a positive difference in the life of any ill or injured person to whom you give aid.

This manual discusses what to do for the common, mild, serious, and life-threatening situations you may face, in a step-by-step-manner, using illustrations and photographs to help you understand the problem at hand. Although it is designed to provide you with a good knowledge base, it is strongly encouraged that you also take a formal first aid course from an organization in your community that provides such training. These organizations include the American Red Cross, the American Heart Association, EMS agencies, and local hospitals. It is also recommended that you refresh your skills on a regular basis.

On behalf of ACEP and emergency medicine specialists throughout the United States, it is my pleasure to bring this fifth edition of the ACEP First Aid Manual to you. I hope that you will enjoy learning how to help those in need of emergency care and that you will gain confidence in your knowledge and skills as you proceed through the book.

Thanks for joining the emergency care team—you can make a difference!

Gina M. Piazza, DO, FACEP
Medical Editor-in-Chief

CONTENTS

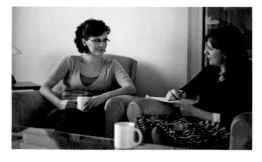

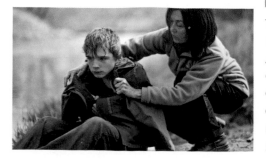

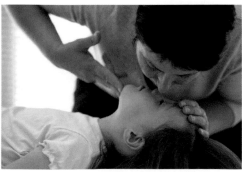

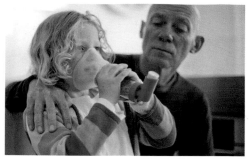

6 WOUNDS AND CIRCULATION 106

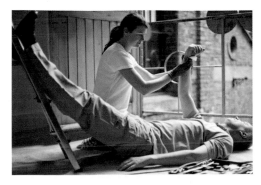

7 BONE, JOINT, AND MUSCLE INJURIES 130

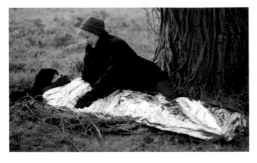

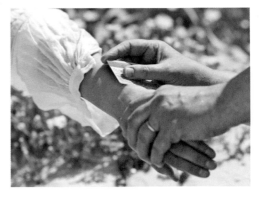

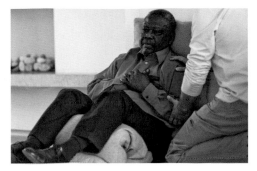

11 TECHNIQUES AND EQUIPMENT 230

12 EMERGENCY FIRST AID 254

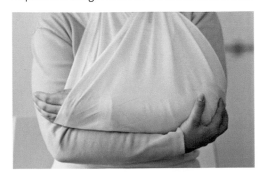

INTRODUCTION

This manual, now in its fifth edition, is published in collaboration with the American College of Emergency Physicians (ACEP). The content is based upon guidelines of the American Heart Association and the American Red Cross. ACEP makes every effort to ensure that its reviewers are knowledgeable content experts. Readers are nevertheless advised that the statements and opinions in this publication are recommendations at the time of publication and should not be construed as official ACEP policy nor should the materials contained here be regarded as a substitute for medical advice. ACEP is not responsible for, and expressly disclaims all liability for, damages of any kind arising out of use, reference to, reliance on, or performance of such information. The materials contained herein are not intended to establish policy, procedure, or a standard of care. First aiders are advised to obtain training from a qualified trainer and keep their certification current, and to recognize the limits of their competence.

The first three chapters provide background information to help you manage a situation safely and learn how to assess a sick or injured person. Treatment for injuries and conditions is given in the chapters that follow, which are grouped by body system or the type of injury. The final chapter provides a quick-reference guide to emergency first aid.

HOW TO USE THIS BOOK

ANATOMY

The chapters are grouped by body system or cause of injury. Within the sections there are easy-to-understand anatomy features that explain the risks involved with particular injuries or conditions and how and why first aid can help.

Color-coded chapters help you find relevant sections easily

Introduction gives an overview of the anatomy for the section

Clear, computer-generated artworks of body systems illustrate each section

Additional artworks provide extra information

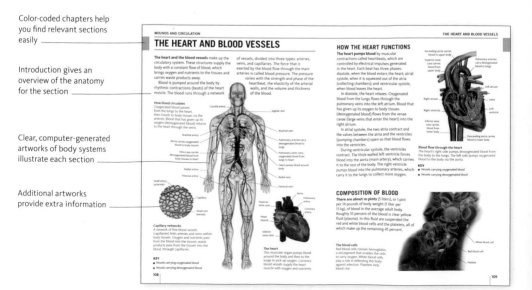

CONDITIONS AND INJURIES

The main part of the book features eight color-coded chapters outlining first aid for more than 110 conditions or injuries. For each entry, there is an introduction that describe the risks and likely cause, then first aid treatment is shown in clear step-by-step instructions.

Introductory text describes background and effects of each condition

Caution boxes alert you to potential risks or alternative treatments

Lists of recognition features help you identify a condition

Your Aims boxes summarize purpose of first aid

Special Case boxes highlight instances where alternative action may be required

Step-by-step instructions explain each stage of treatment

See also references direct you to related conditions

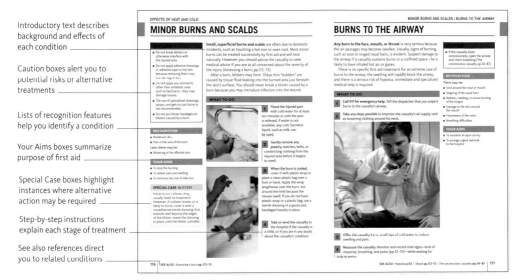

EMERGENCY ADVICE

At the back of the manual is a quick-reference emergency section that provides additional at-a-glance action plans for potentially life-threatening injuries and conditions from unconsciousness and bleeding to asthma and heart attack.

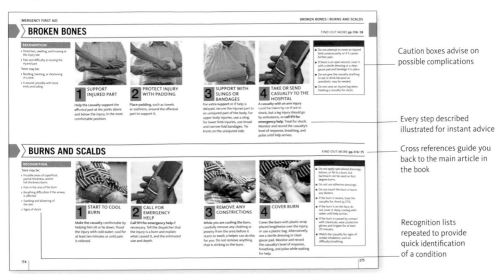

Caution boxes advise on possible complications

Every step described illustrated for instant advice

Cross references guide you back to the main article in the book

Recognition lists repeated to provide quick identification of a condition

1

First aid is the initial assistance or treatment given to a person who is injured or suddenly becomes ill. The person who provides this help may be a first aider, a first responder, a policeman or fireman, or a paramedic or EMT. This chapter prepares you for being a first aider, psychologically and emotionally, as well as giving practical advice on what you should and should not do in an emergency situation.

The information given throughout this book will help you give effective first aid to any casualty in any situation. However, to become a fully competent first aider, you should complete a recognized first aid course and receive certification. This will also strengthen your skills and increase your confidence. The American Red Cross and the American Heart Association teach a variety of first aid courses, at different educational levels.

AIMS AND OBJECTIVES

- To understand your own abilities and limitations.
- To stay safe and calm at all times.
- To assess a situation quickly and calmly and summon the appropriate help if necessary.
- To assist the casualty and provide the necessary treatment, with the help of others if possible.
- To pass on relevant information to the emergency services, or to the person who takes responsibility for the casualty.
- To be aware of your own needs.

BECOMING A FIRST AIDER

WHAT IS A FIRST AIDER?

First aid refers to the actions taken in response to someone who is injured or has suddenly become ill. A first aider is a person who takes action while taking care to keep everyone involved safe (p.28) and to cause no further harm while doing so. Follow the actions that most benefit the casualty, taking into account your own skills, knowledge, and experience, using the guidelines set out in this book.

This chapter prepares you for the role of first aider by providing guidance on responding to a first aid situation and assessing the priorities for the casualty. There is advice on the psychological aspect of giving first aid and practical guidance on how to protect yourself and the casualty.

Chapter 2, Managing an Incident (pp.26–37), provides guidelines on dealing with events (traffic accidents or fires, for example). Chapter 3, Assessing a Casualty (pp.38–53), looks at the practical steps to take when assessing a sick or injured person's condition.

One of the primary rules of first aid is to ensure that an area is safe for you before you approach a casualty (p.28). Do not attempt heroic rescues in hazardous circumstances. If you put yourself at risk, you are unlikely to be able to help casualties and could become one yourself and cause harm to others. If it is not safe, do not approach the casualty, but call 911 for emergency help.

FIRST AID PRIORITIES

- **Assess a situation** quickly and calmly.
- **Protect yourself** and any casualties from danger—never put yourself at risk (p.28).
- **Prevent cross-contamination** between yourself and the casualty as best as possible (p.16).
- **Comfort and reassure** casualties.
- **Assess the casualty:** identify, as best as you can, the injury or nature of illness affecting a casualty (pp.38–53).
- **Give early treatment,** and treat the casualties with the most serious (life-threatening) conditions first.
- **Arrange for appropriate help: call 911 for emergency help** if you suspect serious injury or illness; take or send the casualty to the hospital; transfer him into the care of a healthcare professional, or to a higher level of medical care. Stay with a casualty until care is available.

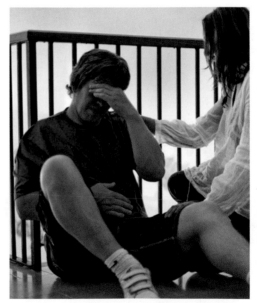

Assessing an incident
When you come across an incident stay calm and support the casualty. Ask him what has happened. Try not to move the casualty; if possible, treat him in the position you find him.

HOW TO PREPARE YOURSELF

When responding to an emergency you should recognize the emotional and physical needs of all involved, including your own. You should look after your own psychological health and be able to recognize stress if it develops (pp.24–25).

A calm, considerate response from you that engenders trust and respect from those around you is fundamental to your being able to give or receive information from a casualty or witnesses effectively. This includes being aware of, and managing, your reactions, so that you can focus on the casualty and make an assessment. By talking to a casualty in a kind, considerate, gentle but firm manner, you will inspire confidence in your actions and this will generate trust between you and the casualty.

Without this confidence he may not tell you about an important event, injury, or symptom, and may remain in a highly distressed state.

The actions described in this chapter aim to help you facilitate this trust, minimize distress, and provide support to promote the casualty's ability to cope and recover. The key steps to being an effective first aider are:

- **Be calm** in your approach
- **Be aware of risks** (to yourself and others)
- **Build and maintain trust** (from the casualty and the bystanders)
- **Give early treatment,** treating the most serious (life-threatening) conditions first
- **Call appropriate help**
- **Remember your own needs**

BE CALM

It is important to be calm in your approach to providing first aid. Consider what situations might challenge you, and how you would deal with them. In order to convey confidence to others and encourage them to trust you, you need to control your own emotions and reactions.

People often fear the unknown. Becoming more familiar with first aid priorities and the key techniques in this book can help you feel more comfortable. By identifying your fears in advance, you can take steps to overcome them. Learn as much as you can, for example, by enrolling in a first aid course, asking others how they dealt with similar situations, or talking your fears through with a person you trust.

STAY IN CONTROL

In an emergency situation, the body responds by releasing hormones that may cause a "fight, flight, or freeze" response. When this happens, your heart beats faster, your breathing quickens, and you may sweat more. You may also feel more alert, want to run away or feel frozen to the spot.

If you feel overwhelmed and slightly panicky, you may feel pressured to do something before you are clear about what is needed. Pause and take a few slow breaths. Consider who else might help you feel calmer, and remind yourself of the first aid priorities (opposite). If you still feel overwhelmed, take another breath and tell yourself to be calmer. When you are calm, you will be better able to think more clearly and plan your response.

The thoughts you have are linked to the way you behave and the way you feel. If you think that you cannot cope, you will have more trouble determining what to do and will feel more anxious: more ready to fight, flee, or freeze. If you know how to calm yourself, you will be better able to deal with anxiety and help the casualty.

PROTECTION FROM INFECTION

When you give first aid, it is important to protect yourself (and the casualty) from infection as well as injury. Take steps to avoid cross-contamination—transmitting germs or infection to a casualty or contracting infection from a casualty. Remember, infection is a risk even with relatively minor injuries. It is a particular concern if you are treating a wound, because blood-borne viruses, such as hepatitis B or C and Human Immunodeficiency Virus (HIV), may be transmitted by contact with blood. In practice, the risk is low and should not deter you from carrying out first aid. The risk increases if an infected person's blood makes contact with yours through a cut or scrape.

Usually, taking measures such as washing your hands and wearing disposable gloves will provide sufficient protection for you and the casualty. There is no known evidence of these blood-borne viruses being transmitted during resuscitation. If a face shield or pocket mask is available, it should be used when you give rescue breaths (pp.68–69 and pp.78–79).

WHEN TO SEEK MEDICAL ADVICE

Take care not to prick yourself with any needle found on or near a casualty, or cut yourself on glass. If you accidentally prick or cut your skin, or splash your eye, wash the area thoroughly and seek medical help immediately. If you are providing first aid on a regular basis, it is advisable to seek guidance on additional personal protection, such as immunization. If you think you have been exposed to an infection while giving first aid, seek medical advice as soon as possible.

CAUTION

To help protect yourself from infection you can carry protective equipment such as:

- Pocket mask or face shield
- Latex-free disposable gloves
- Alcohol gel to clean your hands

MINIMIZING THE RISK OF CROSS-CONTAMINATION

- **Do** wash your hands and wear latex-free disposable gloves (in case you or the casualty are allergic to latex). If gloves are not available, ask the casualty to dress his or her own wound, or enclose your hands in clean plastic bags.
- **Do** cover cuts and scrapes on your hands with waterproof dressings.
- **Do** wear a plastic apron if dealing with large quantities of body fluids, and wear glasses or goggles to protect your eyes.
- **Do** dispose of all waste safely (p.18).
- **Do not** touch a wound or any part of a dressing that will come into contact with a wound with your bare hands.
- **Do not** breathe, cough, or sneeze over a wound while you are treating a casualty.

THOROUGH HAND-WASHING

If you can, **wash your hands** before you touch a casualty, but if this is not possible, wash them as soon as possible afterward. For a thorough wash, pay attention to all parts of the hands— palms, wrists, fingers and thumbs, and fingernails. Use soap and water if available, or rub your hands with alcohol gel.

HOW TO WASH YOUR HANDS

1 **Wet your hands** under running water. Put some soap into the palm of a cupped hand. Rub the palms of your hands together.

2 **Rub the palm** of your left hand against the back of your right hand, then rub the right palm on the back of your left hand.

3 **Interlock the fingers** of both hands and work the soap between them.

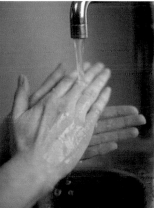
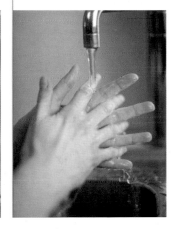

4 **Rub the back** of the fingers of your right hand against the palm of your left hand, then repeat with your left hand in your right palm.

5 **Rub your right thumb** in the palm of your left hand, then your left thumb in the right palm.

6 **Rub the fingertips** of your left hand in the palm of your right hand and vice versa. Rinse thoroughly, then pat dry with a disposable paper towel.

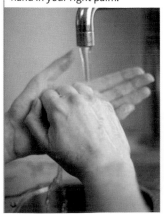
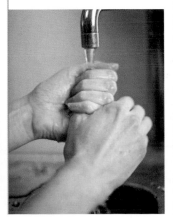
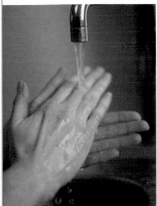

❮❮ PROTECTION FROM INFECTION

USING PROTECTIVE GLOVES

In addition to hand washing, gloves give added protection against infection in a first aid situation. If possible, carry protective, disposable, latex-free gloves with you at all times. Wear them whenever there is a likelihood of contact with blood or other body fluids. If in doubt, wear them anyway.

Disposable gloves should be used to treat only one casualty. Put them on just before you approach a casualty and remove them as soon as the treatment is completed and before you do anything else.

> **CAUTION**
>
> Always use latex-free gloves. Some people have a serious allergy to latex, and this may cause anaphylactic shock (p.223). Nitrile gloves (often blue or purple) are recommended.

When taking off the gloves, hold the top edge of one glove with your other gloved hand and peel it off so that it is inside out. Repeat with the other hand without touching the outside of the gloves. Dispose of them in a biohazard bag (below).

PUTTING ON GLOVES

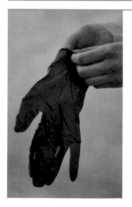

1 **Ideally, wash your hands** before putting on the gloves. Hold one glove by the top and pull it on. Do not touch the main part of the glove with your fingers.

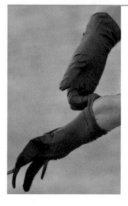

2 **Pick up the second glove** with the gloved hand. With your fingers under the top edge, pull it onto your hand. Your gloved fingers should not touch your skin.

DEALING WITH WASTE

Once you have treated a casualty, all soiled material must be disposed of carefully to prevent the spread of infection.

Place items such as dressings or gloves in a plastic bag—ideally a biohazard bag—and give it to the emergency services. Seal the bag tightly and label it to show that it contains clinical waste. Put sharp objects, including needles, in a plastic container known as a sharps container, which is usually red. If no sharps container is available, put used needles in a jar with a screw top and give it to the EMT for disposal.

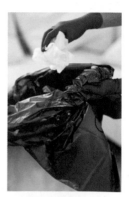

BIOHAZARD BAG

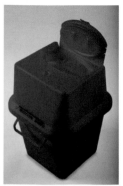

SHARPS CONTAINER

DEALING WITH A CASUALTY

Casualties are often frightened because of what is happening to them, and what may happen next. Your role is to stay calm and take charge of the situation—but be ready to stand back if there is someone better qualified. If there is more than one casualty, use the primary survey (pp.44–45) to identify the most seriously injured casualties and treat in the order of priority.

BUILDING TRUST

Establish trust with your casualty by introducing yourself. Find out what the person likes to be called, and use his name when you talk to him. Crouch or kneel down so that you are at the same height as the casualty. Explain what is happening and why. You will inspire trust if you say what you are doing before you do it. Treat the casualty with dignity and respect at all times. If possible, give him choices, for example, whether he would prefer to sit or lie down and/or who he would like to have with him. Also, if possible, gain his consent before you treat him by asking if he agrees with whatever you are going to do.

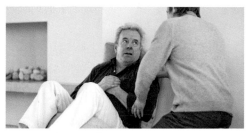

Reassure the casualty
When treating a casualty, remain calm and do not do anything without explanation. Try to answer any questions he may have honestly.

DIVERSITY AND COMMUNICATION

Consider the age and appearance of your casualty when you talk to him, since different people need different responses. Respect people's wishes; accept that someone might want to be treated in a particular way. Communication can be difficult if a person speaks a different language or cannot hear you. Use simple language or signs or write questions down. Ask if anyone speaks the same language as the casualty or knows the person or saw the incident and can describe what happened.

SPECIAL CASE TREATING CHILDREN

You will need to use simpler, shorter words when talking to children. If possible, make sure a child's parents or caregivers are with him, and keep them involved at all times. It is important to establish the caregiver's trust as well as the child's. Talk first to the parent/caregiver and get his or her permission to continue to treat the child. Once the parent/caregiver trusts you, the child will also feel more confident.

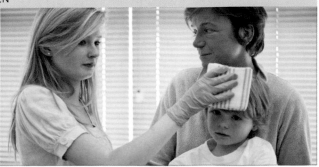

« DEALING WITH A CASUALTY

LISTEN CAREFULLY

Use your eyes and ears to be aware of how a casualty responds. Listen by showing verbal and nonverbal listening skills.

- **Make eye contact,** but look away now and then so as not to stare.
- **Use a calm, confident voice** that is loud enough to be heard but do not shout.
- **Do not speak too quickly.**
- **Keep instructions simple:** use short sentences and simple words.
- **Use affirming nods** and "mmms" to show you are listening when the casualty speaks.
- **Check that the casualty understands** what you mean—ask to make sure.
- **Use simple hand gestures** and movements.
- **Do not interrupt the casualty,** but always acknowledge what you are told; for example, summarize what a casualty has told you to show that you understand.

WHEN A CASUALTY RESISTS HELP

If someone is ill or injured he may be upset, confused, tearful, angry, and/or anxious to get away. Be sensitive to a casualty's feelings; let him know that his reactions are understandable. Also accept that you may not be able to help, or might even be seen as a threat. Stay at a safe distance until you have gained the person's consent to move closer, so that he does not feel crowded. Do not argue or disagree. A casualty may refuse help, for example because he is suffering from a head injury or hypothermia. If you think a person needs something other than what he asks for, explain why. For example, you could say, "I think someone should look at where you're hurt before you move, in case moving makes it worse." If someone still refuses your help and you think he needs urgent medical attention, call 911 for emergency help. A casualty has the right to refuse help, even if it causes further harm. Tell the dispatcher that you have offered first aid and have been refused. If you are worried that a person's condition is deteriorating, observe from a distance until help arrives.

TREATING THE CASUALTY

When treating a casualty, always relate to him calmly and thoughtfully to maintain trust. Think about how he might be feeling. Check that you have understood what the casualty said and consider the impact of your actions, for example, is the casualty becoming more (or less) upset, angry, and tense? A change in emotional state can indicate that a condition is worsening.

Be prepared to change your manner, depending on what a person feels comfortable with; for example, ask fewer questions or talk about something else. Keep a casualty updated and give him options rather than telling him what to do. Ask the casualty about his next-of-kin or friends who can help, and help him make contact with them. Ask if you can help make arrangements so that any responsibilities the casualty may have can be taken care of.

Stay with the casualty. Do not leave someone who may be dying, seriously ill, or badly injured alone except to go to call for emergency help. Talk to the casualty while touching his shoulder or arm, or holding a hand. Never allow a casualty to feel alone.

ENLISTING HELP FROM OTHERS

In an emergency situation you may be faced with several tasks at once: to maintain safety, to call for help, and to start giving first aid. Some of the people at the scene may be able to help you do the following:

- **Make the area safe;** for example, control traffic and keep onlookers away.
- **Call 911 for emergency help** (p.23).
- **Obtain first aid equipment,** for example an AED (automated external defibrillator).
- **Control bleeding** with direct pressure, or support an injured limb.
- **Help maintain the casualty's privacy** by holding a blanket around the scene and encouraging onlookers to move away.
- **Transport the casualty** to a safe place if his life is in immediate danger, only if it is safer to move him than to leave him where he is, and you have the necessary help and equipment (p.234).

The reactions of bystanders may cause you concern or anger. They may have had no first aid training and feel helpless or frightened themselves. If they have seen or been involved in the incident, they too may be injured and distressed. Bear this in mind if you need to ask a bystander to help you. Talk to people in a firm but gentle manner. By staying calm yourself, you will gain their trust and help them remain calm too.

CARE OF PERSONAL BELONGINGS

Make sure the casualty's belongings are with him at all times. If you have to search belongings for identification or clues to a person's condition (medication, for example), do so in front of a reliable witness. If possible, ask the casualty's permission before you do this. Afterward, ensure that all of the clothing and personal belongings and medication accompany the casualty to the hospital or are handed over to the police.

KEEPING NOTES

As you gather information about a casualty, write it down so that you can refer to it later. A written record of the timing of events is particularly valuable to medical personnel. Note, for example, the length of a period of unconsciousness, the duration of a seizure, the time of any changes in the casualty's condition, and the time of any intervention or treatment. Hand your notes to the emergency services when they arrive, or give them to the casualty. Useful information to provide includes:

- **Casualty's details,** including his name, age and contact details
- **History** of the incident or illness
- **Brief description** of any injuries
- **Unusual behavior,** or a change in behavior
- **Treatment**—where given and when
- **Vital signs—level** of response, breathing rate, and pulse (pp.52–53), if the first aider is trained
- **Medical history**
- **Medication** the casualty has taken, with details of the amounts taken and when
- **Next-of-kin** contact details
- **Your contact details** as well as the date, time, and place of your involvement

Remember that any information you gather is confidential. Never share it with anyone not involved in the casualty's care without his agreement. Let the casualty know why you are recording information and who you will give it to. When you are asking for such information, be sensitive to who is around and of the casualty's privacy and dignity.

REQUESTING HELP

Further help is available from a range of sources. If help is needed, you must decide both on the type of help and how to access it. First, carry out a primary survey (pp.44–45) to ascertain the severity of the casualty's condition. If it is not serious, explain the options and allow him to choose where to go. If a casualty's condition is serious, seek emergency help. Throughout the book there are guidelines for choosing the appropriate level of help.

■ **Call 911 for emergency help** if the casualty needs urgent medical attention and should be transported to the hospital in an ambulance, for example, when you suspect a heart attack.

■ **Take or send the casualty to a hospital.** Choose this option when a casualty needs hospital treatment, but his condition is unlikely to worsen; for example, with a finger injury. You can take him yourself if you can arrange transportation—either in your own car or in a taxi.

■ **Seek medical advice.** Depending on what is available in his area, the casualty should be advised to call his own physician or nurse practitioner. He would do this, for example, when he has symptoms such as earache or diarrhea.

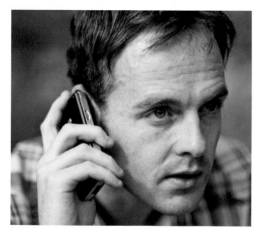

Calling for help
When calling for help in an emergency, stay calm. Be clear and concise and give as much detail as possible.

CALLING FOR HELP

You can call for help from:
■ **Emergency services,** including police, fire and ambulance services, by calling 911
■ **Utilities,** including gas, electricity or water—the phone number will be in the telephone directory
■ **Health services,** including doctor, dentist, and hospital—this varies in different areas. The phone numbers will be in the telephone directory
   Calls to the emergency services are free from any phone, including cell phones. On some roadways, emergency phones have been placed at regular intervals to enable people to

call for help. To summon help using these telephones, pick up the receiver and your call will be answered. However, the density of these phones can vary widely by state and area. You may do better with a cell phone than these highway phones.
   Keep time away from the casualty to a minimum. Ideally, tell someone else to make the call for you while you stay with the casualty. Ask the person to confirm that the call has been made and that help is on the way. If you have to leave a casualty to call for help, first take any necessary vital action (primary survey pp.44–45).

MAKING THE CALL

When you dial 911, you will be asked which service you require. If there are casualties, ask for the ambulance service (EMS); the dispatcher will alert other services if they are required. Always remain on the telephone and let the dispatcher hang up first, because you may be given important information about what to do for the casualty while you wait, and/or asked for further information as the situation develops. If someone else makes the call, make sure that he is aware of the importance of his call and that he reports back to you after making the call.

TALKING TO THE EMERGENCY SERVICES

State your name clearly and say that you are acting in your capacity as a first aider. It is essential to provide the following:

- **Your telephone number** and/or the number you are calling from.
- **The exact location** of the incident; give a road name or number. It can also be helpful to mention any intersections or other landmarks in the area. In many cases your call can be traced if you are unsure of your exact location. If you are on a highway, say in which direction the vehicles were traveling.
- **The type and gravity** of the emergency. For example, "Traffic accident, two cars, road blocked, three people trapped."
- **Number, gender, and age** of casualties. For example, "One man, early sixties, breathing difficulties, suspected heart attack."
- **Details of any hazards,** such as gas, toxic substances, power-line damage, or adverse weather conditions, such as fog or ice.

WHEN THE EMERGENCY SERVICES ARRIVE

Once the emergency services arrive, they will take over the care of the casualty. Tell them what has happened and any treatment given. Hand over any notes you made while attending the casualty. You may be asked to continue helping, for example, by assisting relatives or friends of the casualty while the paramedics provide emergency care.

You should also follow instructions given to you by the medical team. Remain until you are told you can go, since they may need to ask you more questions or the police may want to speak to you. Help maintain a clear and clean environment and preserve the dignity and confidentiality of those involved.

You may be asked to contact a relative. Explain as simply and honestly as you can what has happenened and where the casualty has been taken. Do not be vague or exaggerate because this may cause unnecessary alarm. It is better to admit ignorance than to give someone misleading information.

However, the information you give may cause distress; if so, remain calm and be clear about what to do next.

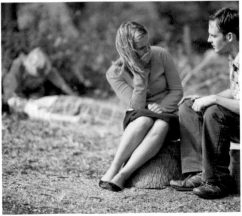

Assisting at the scene
Once the emergency services arrive, tell them everything you know. While they assess and treat the casualty, you may be asked to look after or reassure friends.

THE USE OF MEDICATION

In first aid, administering medication is largely confined to relieving general aches and pains. It usually involves helping a casualty take his own medicines.

A variety of medications can be bought without a doctor's prescription. However, you must not buy or borrow medication to administer to a casualty, or give your own.

If you advise the casualty to take any medication other than that stipulated in this manual, he may be put at risk and you could face legal action as a consequence. Whenever a casualty takes medication, it is essential to make sure that:

- **It is for** the condition
- **It is not out of date**
- **It is taken as advised**
- **Any precautions** are strictly followed
- **The recommended dose** is not exceeded
- **You keep a record** of the name and dose of the medication as well as the time and method of administration

> **CAUTION**
>
> Aspirin should never be given to anyone under the age of 16 years because there is risk of a rare condition called Reye's syndrome.

REMEMBER YOUR OWN NEEDS

Most people who learn first aid gain significantly from doing so. In addition to learning new skills and meeting new people, by learning first aid you can make a real difference in peoples' lives. Being able to help people who are ill or injured often results in a range of positive feelings. However, you may also feel stressed when you are called upon to administer first aid, and feel emotional once you have finished treating a casualty, whatever the outcome. Occasionally, that stress can interfere with your physical and mental well-being after an incident. Everyone responds to stressful situations in different ways, and some people are more susceptible to stress than others. It is important to learn how to deal with any stress in order to maintain your own health and effectiveness as a first aider. Gaining an understanding of your own needs can help you be better prepared for future situations.

IMMEDIATELY AFTER AN INCIDENT

An emergency is an emotional experience. Many first aiders experience satisfaction, or even elation, and most cope well. However, after you have treated a casualty, depending on the type of incident and the outcome, you might experience a mixture of the following:

- Satisfaction
- Confusion, worry, doubt
- Anger, sadness, fear

You may go through what has happened again and again in your mind, so it can be helpful to talk to someone you trust about how you feel and what you did. Consider talking to someone else who was there, or who you know has had a similar experience. Never reproach yourself or hide your feelings. This is especially important if the outcome was not as you had hoped. Even with appropriate treatment, and however hard you try, a casualty may not recover.

LATER REACTIONS

Delivering first aid can lead to positive feelings because you notice new things about yourself, such as your ability to deal with a crisis. However, occasionally, the effect of an incident on you will depend on your first aid experience as well as on the nature of the actual incident.

The majority of the incidents you will deal with will be of a minor nature and they will probably involve people you know. If you have witnessed an incident that involved a threat to life or you have experienced a feeling of helplessness, you may find yourself suffering from feelings of stress after the incident. In most cases, these feelings will disappear over time.

WHEN TO SEEK HELP

If, however, you experience persistent or distressing symptoms associated with a stressful incident, such as nightmares and flashbacks, seek further help from someone you trust and feel you can confide in.

See your doctor or a mental health professional if you feel overwhelmed by your symptoms. You can talk through them with the professionals and together decide what is best for you. Seeking help is nothing to be embarrassed about, and it is important to overcome these feelings. This will not only help you deal with your current reactions, but it will also help you learn how to respond to situations in the future.

Talking things over

Confiding in a friend or relative is often useful. Ideally, talk to someone who was also present at the incident; she may have the same feelings about it as you. If you are unable to deal with the effects of the event you were part of or witnessed, seek help from your doctor.

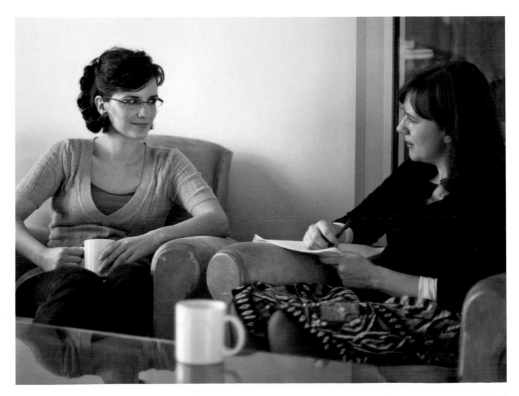

2

The scene of any incident can present many potential dangers, whether someone has become ill or has been injured, whether in the home or outside at the scene of an incident. Before any first aid is provided you must make sure that approaching the scene of the incident does not present unacceptable danger to the casualty, or to you or anyone else who is helping.

This chapter provides advice for first aiders on how to ensure safety in an emergency situation. There are specific guidelines for emergencies that pose a particular risk. These include fires, traffic accidents, and incidents involving electricity and drowning.

The procedures that are used by the emergency services for major incidents, where particular precautions are necessary and where first aiders may be called on to help, are also described here.

AIMS AND OBJECTIVES

- To protect yourself from danger and make the area safe.
- To assess the situation quickly and calmly and summon help if necessary.
- To assist any casualties and provide necessary treatment with the help of bystanders.
- To call 911 for emergency help if you suspect serious injury or illness.
- To be aware of your own needs.

MANAGING
AN INCIDENT

ACTION AT AN EMERGENCY

In any emergency it is important that you follow a clear plan of action. This will enable you to prioritize the demands that may be made upon you, and help you decide on your best response.

The principle steps are: to assess the situation, to make the area safe (if possible), and to give first aid. Use the primary survey (pp.44–45) to identify the most seriously injured casualties and treat them in the order of priority.

ASSESSING THE SITUATION

Evaluating the scene accurately is one of the most important factors in the management of an incident. You should stay calm. State that you have first aid training and, if there are no medical personnel in attendance, calmly take charge.

Identify any safety risks and assess the resources available. Action for key dangers you may face, such as fire, are dealt with in this chapter, but be aware, too, of tripping hazards, sharp objects, chemical spills, and falling debris.

All incidents should be managed in a similar manner. Consider the following:

- **Safety** What are the dangers and do they still exist? Are you wearing protective equipment? Is it safe for you to approach?
- **Scene** What factors are involved at the incident? What are the mechanisms of the injuries (pp.42–43)? How many casualties are there? What are the potential injuries?
- **Situation** What happened? How many people are involved and what ages are they? Are any of them children or elderly?

MAKING AN AREA SAFE

The conditions that give rise to an incident may still present a danger and must be eliminated if possible. It may be that a simple measure, such as turning off the ignition of a car to reduce the risk of fire, is sufficient. As a last resort, move the casualty to safety. Usually specialist help and equipment is required for this.

When approaching a casualty, make sure you protect yourself: wear high-visibility clothing, gloves, and head protection if you have them. Remember, too, that a casualty faces the risk of injury from the same hazards that you face. If extrication from the scene is delayed, try to protect the casualty from any additional hazards.

If you cannot make an area safe, **call 911 for emergency help** before performing first aid. Stand clear until the emergency services have secured the scene.

GIVING EMERGENCY HELP

Once an area has been made safe, use the primary survey (pp.44–45) to quickly carry out an initial assessment of the casualty or casualties to establish treatment priorities. If there is more than one casualty, attend to those

with life-threatening conditions first. If possible, treat casualties in the position in which you find them; move them only if they are in immediate danger or if it is necessary in order to provide life-saving treatment. Enlist help from others if possible. Ask bystanders to call for the emergency services (p.23). They can also help protect a casualty's privacy, put out flares or warning triangles in the event of a vehicle accident (p.30), or retrieve equipment while you begin first aid.

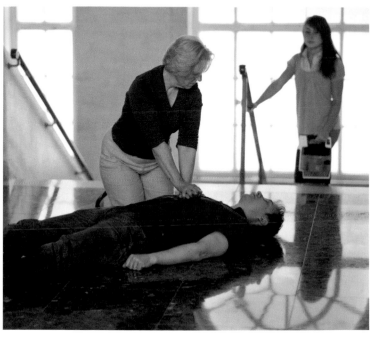

Begin treatment
Start life-saving first aid as soon as possible. Ask others to call for help and retrieve equipment such as an AED (automated external defibrillator).

ASSISTING THE EMERGENCY SERVICES

Hand over any notes you have made to the emergency services when they arrive (p.21). Answer any questions they may have and follow any instructions. As a first aider you may be asked to help, for example, to move a casualty using specialist equipment. If so, you should always follow their instructions.

HELICOPTER RESCUE

Occasionally, helicopter rescue is required. If a casualty is being rescued in this way, there are a number of safety rules to follow. If the emergency services are already present, you should stay clear unless they give you specific instructions.

If the emergency services are not present, keep bystanders clear. Make sure everyone is at least 50 yards (45 meters) away, and that no one is smoking. Kneel down as the helicopter approaches, keeping well away from the rotor blades. Once it has landed, do not approach it. Keep bystanders back and wait for a member of the crew to approach you.

TRAFFIC ACCIDENTS

The severity of traffic accidents can range from a fall from a bicycle to a major vehicle crash involving many casualties. Often, the accident site will present serious risks to safety, largely because of passing traffic.

It is essential to make the accident area safe before attending any casualties (p.28); this protects you, the casualties, and other road users. Once the area is safe, quickly assess the casualties and prioritize treatment. Give first aid to those with life-threatening injuries before treating anyone else. **Call 911 for emergency help,** giving as much detail as you can about the accident, indicating number and age of the casualties, and types of injury.

MAKING THE ACCIDENT AREA SAFE

Do not put yourself or others in further danger. Take the following precautions:

- **Park safely,** well away from the site of the accident, set your hazard lights flashing, and put on a high-visibility jacket/vest if you have one.
- **Set up warning triangles** or flares (or position another vehicle that has hazard lights) at least 50 yards (45 meters) from the accident in each direction; bystanders can do this while you attend to the casualty. If possible, send helpers to warn oncoming drivers to slow down.

- **Make vehicles safe.** For example, switch off the ignition of any damaged vehicle. Stabilize vehicles. If a vehicle is upright, and you can get in without risk to yourself, apply the emergency brake, put it in park, or place blocks in front of the wheels. If it is on its side, do not attempt to right it.
- **Watch out for physical dangers,** such as traffic. Make sure that no one smokes anywhere near the accident.
- **Alert the emergency services** to damaged power lines, fuel spills, or any vehicles with HAZMAT signs (opposite).

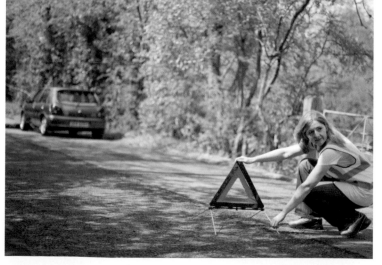

Warn other road users
Ask a bystander to set up warning triangles in both directions. Advise the person to watch for other vehicles while she is doing this.

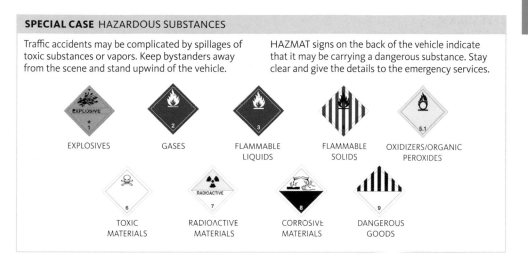

SPECIAL CASE HAZARDOUS SUBSTANCES

Traffic accidents may be complicated by spillages of toxic substances or vapors. Keep bystanders away from the scene and stand upwind of the vehicle.

HAZMAT signs on the back of the vehicle indicate that it may be carrying a dangerous substance. Stay clear and give the details to the emergency services.

EXPLOSIVES   GASES   FLAMMABLE LIQUIDS   FLAMMABLE SOLIDS   OXIDIZERS/ORGANIC PEROXIDES

TOXIC MATERIALS   RADIOACTIVE MATERIALS   CORROSIVE MATERIALS   DANGEROUS GOODS

ASSESSING THE CASUALTIES

Quickly assess any casualties by carrying out a primary survey (pp.44–45). Deal first with those who have life-threatening injuries. Assume that any casualty who has been involved in a traffic accident may have a neck or spinal injury (pp.157–59). If possible, treat casualties in the position in which you find them, supporting the head and neck at all times, and wait for the emergency services.

Search the area around the accident thoroughly to make sure you do not overlook any casualty who may have been thrown clear, or who has wandered away from the site. Bystanders can help. If a person is trapped in or under a vehicle, she will need to be released by the fire department. Monitor and record the casualty's vital signs—level of response, breathing, and pulse (pp.52–53) if trained—while you wait.

CAUTION

- Do not cross a highway to attend to an accident or casualty.
- At night, wear or carry something light or reflective, such as a high-visibility jacket, and use a flashlight.
- Do not move the casualty unless it is absolutely necessary. If you do have to move her, the method will depend on the casualty's condition and available help.
- Be aware that road surfaces may be slippery because of fuel, oil, or even ice.
- Be aware that undeployed air bags and unactivated seat-belt tensioners may be a hazard.
- Find out as much as you can about the accident and relay this information to the emergency services when they arrive.

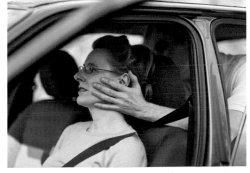

Casualty in a vehicle
Assume that any injured casualty in a vehicle has a neck injury. Support the head while you await help. Reassure her and keep her ears uncovered so that she can hear you.

FIRES

Fire spreads very quickly, so your first priority is to warn any people at risk. If in a building, activate the nearest fire alarm, **call 911 for emergency help,** then leave the building. However, if doing this delays your escape, make the call when you are out of the building. As a first aider, try to keep everyone calm. Encourage and assist people to evacuate the area.

When arriving at an incident involving fire, stop, observe, think: do not enter the area. A minor fire can escalate in minutes to a serious blaze. **Call 911 for emergency help** and wait for it to arrive.

THE ELEMENTS OF FIRE

A fire needs three components to start and maintain it: ignition (a spark or flame); a source of fuel (gasoline, wood, or fabric); and oxygen (air). Removing one of these elements can break this "triangle of fire."

- **Remove combustible materials,** such as paper or cardboard, from the path of a fire, because they can fuel the flames.
- **Cut off a fire's oxygen** supply by shutting a door on a fire or smothering the flames with a fire blanket. This will cause the fire to suffocate and go out.
- **Turn off a car's ignition,** or switch off the gasoline supply.

LEAVING A BURNING BUILDING

If you see or suspect a fire in a building, activate the first fire alarm you see. Try to help people out of the building without putting yourself at risk. Close doors behind you to help prevent the fire from spreading. If you are in a public building, use the fire exits and look for assembly points outside.

You should already know the evacuation procedure at your workplace. If, however, you are visiting other premises you are not familiar with, follow the signs for escape routes and obey any instructions given by the fire marshals.

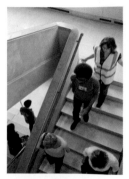

Evacuating other people
Encourage people to leave the building calmly but quickly via the nearest exit. If they have to use the stairs, make sure they do not rush and risk falling down.

CAUTION
When escaping from a fire:
■ Do not reenter a burning building to collect personal possessions
■ Do not use elevators
■ Do not go back to a building unless cleared to do so by a fire officer
Fire precautions:
■ Do not move anything that is on fire
■ Do not smother flames with flammable materials
■ Do not fight a fire if it could endanger your own safety
■ If your clothes catch fire and help is not available, you can extinguish the flames yourself by stopping, dropping to the ground, and rolling
■ Do not put water on an electrical fire: pull the plug out or switch the power off
■ Smother a grease fire with a fire blanket or pot lid; never use water

CLOTHING ON FIRE

Always follow this procedure: Stop, Drop, and Roll.

- **Stop** the casualty from panicking, running around, or going outside; any movement or breeze will fan the flames.
- **Drop** the casualty to the ground. If possible, wrap him tightly in a fire blanket, or heavy fabric such as a coat, curtain, blanket (not a nylon blanket or an openweave type of any material—acrylic, wool, cotton, or other), or rug.
- **Roll** the casualty along the ground until the flames have been smothered. Treat any burns (pp.174–80): help the casualty lie down with the burned side uppermost, and cool the burn by applying cool water or fanning the area gently.

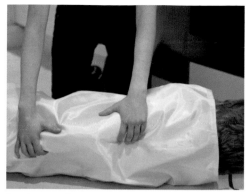

Putting out flames
Help the casualty onto the ground to stop flames from rising to his face. Wrap him in a fire blanket to starve flames of oxygen, and roll him on the ground until the flames are extinguished.

SMOKE AND FUMES

Any fire in a confined space creates a highly dangerous atmosphere that is low in oxygen and may also be polluted by carbon monoxide and other toxic fumes. Never enter a smoke- or fume-filled building or open a door leading to a fire. Let the emergency services do this.

- **If you are trapped** in a burning building, if possible go into a room at the front of the building with a window and shut the door. Block gaps under the door by placing a rug or similar heavy fabric across the bottom of the door to minimize smoke. Open the window and shout for help.
- **Stay low** if you have to cross a smoke-filled room: air is clearest at floor level.
- **If escaping** through a high window, climb out backward feet first and lower yourself to the full length of your arms before dropping down.

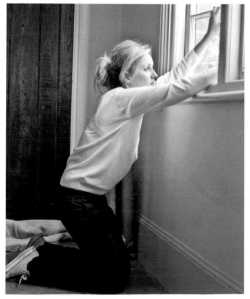

Avoiding smoke and fumes
Shut the door of the room you are in and put a rug or blanket against the door to keep smoke out. Open the window and shout for help. Keep as low as possible to avoid fumes in the room.

ELECTRICAL INCIDENTS

When a person is electrocuted, the passage of electrical current through the body may stun him, causing his breathing and heartbeat to stop. The electrical current can also cause burns both where it enters and where it exits the body to go to "earth." An electrical burn may appear very small or not be visible on the skin, but the damage can extend deep into the tissues (p.178).

Factors that affect the severity of the injury are: the voltage; the type of current; and the path of the current. A low voltage of 110–120 volts is found in most outlets of a home or workplace, but large appliances require 220–240-volt outlets. Industrial outlets may be up to 440 volts. The type of current will either be alternating (AC) or direct (DC), and the path of the current can be hand-to-hand, hand-to-foot, or foot-to-foot.

Most low-voltage and high-tension currents are AC, which causes muscular spasms (tetany) and the "locked-on" phenomenon—the casualty's grasp is "locked" onto the object, preventing him from letting go, so he may remain electrically charged ("live"). In contrast, DC tends to produce a single large muscular contraction that often throws the person away from the source. Be aware that the jolt may cause the casualty to be thrown or to fall, resulting in injuries such as spinal injuries and fractures.

CAUTION

- Do not touch the casualty if he is in contact with the electrical current.

- Do not use anything metallic to break the electrical contact.

- Do not approach high-voltage wires until the power is turned off.

- Do not move a person with an electrical injury unless he is in immediate danger and is no longer in contact with the electricity.

- If it is safe to touch the casualty and he is unconscious and not breathing, start CPR with chest compressions (pp.54–87).

HIGH-VOLTAGE CURRENT

Contact with a high-voltage current found in power lines and overhead cables, is usually immediately fatal. Anyone who survives will have severe burns since the temperature of the electricity may reach up to 9,000°F (5,000°C). Furthermore, the shock produces a muscular spasm that propels the casualty some distance, causing additional injuries.

High-voltage electricity may jump ("arc") up to 20 yards (18 m). The power must be cut off and isolated before the casualty is approached. A casualty who has suffered this type of shock is likely to be unconscious. Once you have been officially informed that it is safe to approach, assess the casualty, and if he is not breathing, begin CPR with chest compressions (pp.54–87).

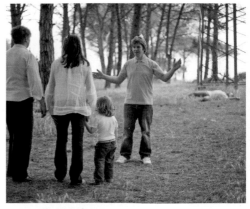

Protect bystanders
Keep everyone away from the incident. Bystanders should stay at least 20 yards (18 m) from the damaged cable and/or casualty.

LOW-VOLTAGE CURRENT

Domestic current, as used in homes and workplaces, can cause serious injury or even death. Incidents are usually due to faulty switches, frayed cords, or defective appliances. Young children are at risk because they are naturally curious, and may put their fingers or other objects into electrical wall sockets.

Water is also a very efficient conductor of electricity, so presents additional risks. Handling an otherwise safe electrical appliance with wet hands, or when you are standing on a wet floor, greatly increases the risk of an electric shock.

BREAKING CONTACT WITH THE ELECTRICITY

1 **Before beginning any treatment,** look first, do not touch. If the casualty is still in contact with the electrical source, he will be "live" and you risk electrocution.

2 **Turn off the source of electricity,** to break the contact between the casualty and the electrical supply. Switch off the current at the circuit box if possible. Otherwise, turn off the electricity at the wall switch, if there is one.

3 **After the power is turned off,** move the source away from both you and the casualty.

4 **Once you are sure that the power is off** and contact between the casualty and the electricity has been broken, perform a primary survey (pp.44–45) and treat any condition found. **Call 911 for emergency help.**

LIGHTNING

A natural burst of electricity discharged from the atmosphere, lightning forms an intense trail of light and heat. Lightning seeks contact with the ground through the nearest tall feature in the landscape and, sometimes, through anyone standing nearby. However, the short duration of a lightning strike usually precludes serious

thermal injury. It may, however, set clothing on fire, knock the casualty down, or cause heart and breathing to stop (cardiac arrest, p.57). Cardiopulmonary resuscitation/CPR (adult, pp.66–71; child, pp.76–79; infant, pp.82–83) must be started promptly. Always clear everyone from the site of a lightning strike since it can strike again in the same place.

WATER INCIDENTS

Incidents around water may involve people of any age. However, drowning is one of the most common causes of accidental death among young people under the age of 16. Young children can drown in fish ponds, paddling pools, bathtubs, and even in buckets or the toilet if they fall in head first, as well as in swimming pools, in the sea, and in open water. Many cases of drowning involve people who have been swimming in strong currents or very cold water, or who have been swimming or boating after drinking alcohol.

There are particular dangers connected with incidents involving swimmers in cold water. The sudden immersion in cold water can result in an overstimulation of nerves, causing the heart to stop (cardiac arrest). Cold water may cause hypothermia (pp.186–87) and exacerbate shock (pp.112–13). Spasm in the throat and inhalation of water can block the airway (hypoxia, p.92, and drowning, p.100). Inhaled or swallowed water may be absorbed into the circulatory system, causing water overload to the brain, heart, or lungs. The exertion of swimming can also strain the heart. Such incidents may happen in the winter, if someone falls through the ice when skating on a pond or pursuing a pet.

> **CAUTION**
>
> - If the casualty is unconscious, lift him out of the water, support his head and neck, and carry him, his head lower than his chest to keep him from inhaling water and protect the airway if he vomits.
> - If removal from the water cannot be immediate, begin rescue breaths while still in the water.
> - When you reach land, check for normal breathing and, if not, begin CPR with compressions (pp.54–87).

WATER RESCUE

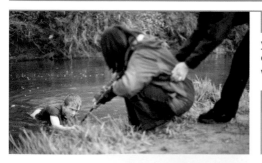

1 **Your first priority** is to get the casualty onto dry land with the minimum of danger to yourself. Stay on dry land, hold out a stick, a branch or a rope for him to grab, then pull him from the water. Alternatively, throw him a float.

2 **If you are a trained lifesaver,** there is no danger to yourself, and the casualty is unconscious, wade or swim to the casualty and tow him ashore. If you cannot do this safely, **call 911 for emergency help.**

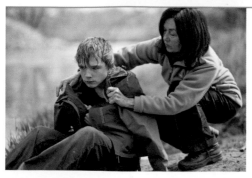

3 **Once the casualty is out of the water,** shield him from the wind, if possible. Treat him for drowning (p.100) and the effects of severe cold (pp.186–88). If possible, replace any wet clothing with dry clothing.

4 **Arrange to take or send** the casualty to the hospital, even if he seems to have recovered completely. If you are at all concerned, **call 911 for emergency help.**

MAJOR INCIDENT/MASS CASUALTIES

A **major incident,** or mass casualty incident, is one that presents a serious threat to the safety of a community, or may cause so many casualties that it requires special arrangements from the emergency services. Events of this kind can overwhelm the resources of the emergency services because there may be more casualties to treat than there are personnel available.

It is the responsibility of the emergency services to declare a situation to be a mass casualty, and certain procedures will be activated by them if necessary. The area around the incident will be sealed off and hospitals and emergency response personnel notified. Organizing this is not a first aider's responsibility, but you may be asked to help.

If you are the first person on the scene of what may be a mass casualty, do not approach it. **Call 911 for emergency help** immediately (pp.22–23). The dispatcher will need to know the type of incident that has occurred (for example, a fire, a traffic accident, or an explosion), the location, the access, any particular hazards and the approximate number of casualties.

EMERGENCY SERVICE SCENE ORGANIZATION

First, the area immediately around the incident will be cordoned off—the inner perimeter. Around this an outer perimeter, the minimum safe area for emergency personnel (fire, ambulance and police), will be established. No one without the correct identification and safety equipment will be allowed inside the area. The on-scene commander, typically the fire chief, will lead the response. Triage of casualties will occur and if the scene is safe and conditions permit, casualties in need of medical treatment will be moved to a casualty collection point.

- **Casualties who cannot walk** will undergo further assessment. They will be assigned to Red / Priority One (immediate) or Yellow / Priority Two (urgent) areas for treatment, and transferred to a hospital by ambulance as soon as possible.
- **Walking casualties** with minor injuries will be assigned to the Green /Priority Three area for treatment and transferred to a hospital if necessary.
- **Uninjured people** may be taken to a survivor reception center.
- **Dead or** critically injured casualties will be assigned to the Gray or Black categories.

TRIAGE

The emergency services use a system called triage to assess casualties. All casualties undergo a primary survey (pp.44–45) at the scene to establish treatment priorities. This will be followed by a secondary survey (pp.46–48) in the casualty collection point. This check will be repeated and any change monitored until a casualty recovers or is transferred into the care of a medical team.

FIRST AIDER'S ROLE

You will not be allowed to enter the perimeter area without adequate personal safety equipment or approval from emergency services personnel. You may be asked to assist the emergency services by, for example, helping identify casualties that have minor injuries, supporting injured limbs, making a note of casualties' names, and/or helping contact their relatives.

3

When a person suddenly becomes ill or has been injured, it is important to find out what is wrong as quickly as possible. However, your first priority is to make sure that you are not endangering yourself by approaching a casualty.

Once you are sure that an incident area is safe, you need to begin your assessment of the casualty or casualties. This chapter explains how to approach each casualty and plan your assessment using a methodical two-stage system, first to check and treat any life-threatening conditions according to their priority (primary survey), then to carry out a detailed assessment looking for injuries that are not immediately apparent (secondary survey). There is advice on deciding treatment priorities, managing more than one casualty, and arranging aftercare. A casualty's condition may improve or deteriorate while in your care, so there is guidance on how to monitor changes in his condition.

AIMS AND OBJECTIVES

- To assess a situation quickly and calmly, while first protecting yourself and the casualty from any danger.
- To assess each casualty and treat life-threatening injuries first.
- To carry out a more detailed assessment of each casualty.
- To seek appropriate help. **Call 911 for emergency help** if you suspect serious injury or illness.
- To be aware of your own needs.

ASSESSING A
CASUALTY

ASSESSING THE SICK OR INJURED

From the previous chapters you now know that to ensure the best possible outcome for anyone who is injured or suddenly becomes ill you need to take responsibility for making assessments. Tell those at the scene that you are a trained first aid provider and calmly take control. However, as indicated in Chapter 2 (pp.26–37), resist the temptation to begin dealing with any casualty until you have the assessed the overall situation, ensured that everyone involved is safe and, if appropriate, taken steps to organize the necessary help. As you read this chapter, look back at Chapter 1 (pp.12–25) and remember the following:

- Be calm
- Be aware of risks
- **Build and maintain** the casualty's trust
- Call appropriate help
- Remember your own needs

MANAGING THE INJURED OR SICK

There are three aspects to this:
- **First,** find out what is wrong with the casualty
- **Second,** treat conditions found in order of severity—life-threatening conditions first
- **Third,** arrange for the next step of a casualty's care. You will need to decide what type of care a casualty needs. You may need to call for emergency help, suggest the casualty seeks medical advice, or allow him to go home, accompanied if you think it is necessary. Other people at the incident can help you with this. **Ask one of them to call 911** for emergency help while you attend a casualty. Alternatively, they may be able to look after less seriously injured casualties, or retrieve first aid equipment.

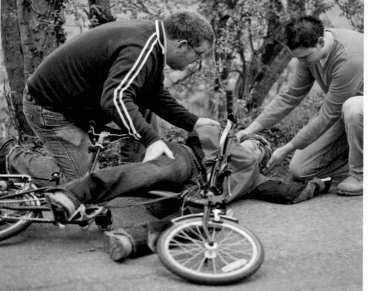

First actions
Support the casualty; a bystander may be able to help. Ask the casualty what happened, and try to identify the most serious injury.

METHODS OF ASSESSMENT

When you assess a casualty you first need to identify and deal with any life-threatening conditions or injuries—the primary survey. Deal with each life-threatening condition as you find it, working in the following order—airway, breathing, circulation—before you progress to the next stage. Depending on your findings, you may not move on to the next stage of the assessment. If the life-threatening injuries are successfully managed, or there are none, you can continue the assessment and perform a secondary survey.

THE PRIMARY SURVEY

This is an initial rapid assessment of a casualty to establish and treat conditions that are an immediate threat to life (pp.44–45).

If a casualty is conscious, suffering from minor injuries and is talking to you, then this survey will be completed very quickly. If, however, a casualty is more seriously injured (for example, unconscious), this assessment will take longer.

Follow the Airway, Breathing, and Circulation (ABC) principle:

- **Airway** Is the airway open and clear? The airway is not open and clear if the casualty is unable to speak. An obstructed airway will prevent breathing, causing hypoxia (p.92) and, ultimately, death. The airway is open and clear if the casualty is talking to you.
- **Breathing** Is the casualty breathing normally? If the casualty is not breathing normally, **call 911 for emergency help**, then start chest compressions with rescue breaths (cardiopulmonary resuscitation/CPR). If this

happens, you are unlikely to move on to the next stage. If the casualty is breathing, check for and treat any breathing difficulty such as asthma, then move on to the next stage: circulation.

- **Circulation** Is the casualty bleeding severely? If he is bleeding this must be treated immediately because it can lead to a life-threatening condition known as shock (pp.112–13). **Call 911 for emergency help.** If there is no bleeding, continue to the secondary survey.

THE SECONDARY SURVEY

This is a detailed examination of a casualty to look for other injuries or conditions that may not be readily apparent on the primary survey (pp.46–48). To do this, carry out a head-to-toe examination (pp.49–51). Your aim is to find out:

- **History** What actually happened and any relevant medical history.
- **Symptoms** Injuries or abnormalities that the casualty tells you about.
- **Signs** Injuries or abnormalities that you can see.

By checking the recognition features of the different injuries and conditions explained in the chapters of this book you can identify what may be wrong. Record your findings and pass on any relevant information to the medical team.

LEVEL OF RESPONSE

You will initially have noted whether or not a casualty is conscious. He may have spoken to you or made eye contact or some other gesture (p.44). Or perhaps there has been no response to your questions such as "Are you all right?" or "What happened?" Now you need to establish the level of response using the AVPU scale (p.52). This is important because some illnesses and injuries cause a deterioration in a casualty's level of response, so it is vital to assess the level, then monitor him for changes.

SPECIAL CASE SEVERAL CASUALTIES

If there is more than one casualty, you will need to prioritize those that must be treated first according to the severity of their injuries. Use the primary survey ABC principles (above) to do this. Remember that unresponsive casualties are at greatest risk.

MECHANISMS OF INJURY

The type of injury that a person sustains is directly related to how the injury is caused. Whether a casualty sustains a single injury or multiple injuries is also determined by the mechanisms that caused it. This is the reason why a history of the incident is important. In many situations, this vital information can be obtained only by those people who deal with the casualty at the scene—often first aiders. Look, too, at the circumstances in which an injury was sustained and the forces that were involved.

The information is useful because it also helps the emergency services and medical team predict the type and severity of injury, as well as the treatment. This therefore helps the diagnosis, treatment, and likely outcome for the casualty.

CIRCUMSTANCES OF INJURY

The extent and type of injuries sustained due to impact—for example, a fall from a height or the impact of a car crash—can be predicted if you know exactly how the incident happened. For example, a car occupant is more likely to sustain serious injuries in a side-impact collision than in a frontal collision at the same speed. This is because the side of the car provides less protection and cannot absorb as much energy as the front of the vehicle. For a driver wearing a seatbelt whose vehicle is struck either head-on or from behind, a specific pattern of injuries can be suspected. The driver's body will be suddenly propelled one way, but the driver's head will lag behind briefly before moving. This results in a "whiplashing" movement of the neck (below). The casualty may also have injuries caused by the seatbelt restraint; for example, fracture of the breastbone and possibly bruising of the heart or lungs. There may be injuries to the face due to contact with the steering wheel or an inflated airbag.

Whiplash
The head may be whipped backward and then rapidly forward, or vice versa, due to sudden forces on the body, such as in a car crash. This produces a whiplash injury, with strained muscles and stretched ligaments in the neck.

FORCES EXERTED ON THE BODY

The energy forces exerted during an impact are another important indicator of the type or severity of any injury. For example, if a man falls from a height of 3 feet (1 m) or less onto hard ground, he will probably suffer bruising but no serious injury. A fall from a height of more than 10 feet (3 m), however, is more likely to produce more serious injuries, such as a pelvic fracture or internal bleeding. An apparently less serious fall can mask a more dangerous injury. A fall from a standing position in susceptible people, like the elderly, those suffering from bone disorders, or those who taking blood thinners, can result in serious head or other injuries.

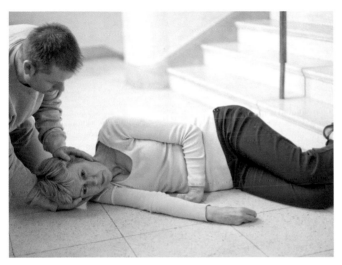

Most serious injury may be hidden
A first aider should keep the casualty still, ask someone to support her head, and **call 911 for emergency help.**

QUESTIONS TO ASK AT THE SCENE

When you are attending a casualty, ask the casualty, or any witnesses, questions to try to find out the mechanism of the injury. Witnesses are especially important if the casualty is unable to talk to you. Possible questions include:
- **Was the casualty ejected from a vehicle?**
- **Was the casualty wearing** a seat belt?
- **Did the vehicle roll over?**
- **Was the casualty wearing a helmet?**
- **How far did the casualty fall?**

- **What type of surface did she land on?**
- **Is there evidence of body contact** with a solid object, such as the floor, a coffee table, or a vehicle's windshield?
- **How did she fall?** (For example, twisting falls can stretch or tear the ligaments or tissues around a joint such as the knee or ankle.)

Pass on all the information that you have gathered to the emergency services (pp.21 and 23).

PRIMARY SURVEY

The primary survey is a quick, systematic assessment of a casualty to establish if any conditions or injuries sustained are life threatening. By following a methodical sequence using established techniques, each life-threatening condition can be identified in a priority order and dealt with on a "find and treat" basis. The sequence should be applied to every casualty you attend. You should not allow yourself to be distracted from it by other events.

The chart opposite guides you through this sequence. Depending on your findings you may not move on to the next stage of the assessment. Only when life-threatening conditions are successfully managed, or there are none, should you perform a secondary survey (pp.46–48).

RESPONSE

At this point you need to make a quick assessment to find out whether a casualty is conscious or unconscious. Observe the casualty as you approach. Introduce yourself even if he does not appear to be responding to you. Ask the casualty some questions, such as, "What happened?" or "Are you all right?" or give a command, such as "Open your eyes!" If there is no initial response, gently shake the casualty's shoulders. If the casualty is a child, tap his shoulder; if he is an infant, tap his foot. If there is still no response, he is unconscious. If the casualty responds and makes eye contact or some other gesture, he is conscious.

Unconscious casualties take priority and require urgent treatment (pp.54–87).

AIRWAY

The first step is to check that a casualty's airway is open and clear. If a casualty is alert and talking to you, it follows that the airway is open and clear. If, however, a casualty is unconscious, the airway may be obstructed (p.59). You need to open and clear the airway (adult, p.63; child, p.73; infant, p.80)—do not move on to the next stage until it is open and clear.

BREATHING

Is the casualty breathing normally? Look, listen, and feel for breaths. If he is alert and/or talking to you, he will be breathing. However, it is important to note the rate, depth, and ease with which he is breathing. For example, conditions such as asthma (p.102) that cause breathing difficulty require urgent treatment.

If an unconscious casualty is not breathing, the heart will stop. Chest compressions and rescue breaths (cardiopulmonary resuscitation/CPR) must be started immediately (adult, pp.66–71; child, pp.76–79; infant, pp.82–83).

CIRCULATION

Conditions that affect the circulation of blood can be life threatening. Injuries that result in severe bleeding (p.114–15) can cause blood loss from the circulatory system, so they must be treated immediately to minimize the risk of a life-threatening condition known as shock (pp.112–13).

Only when life-threatening conditions have been stabilized, or there are none present, should you make a detailed secondary survey of the casualty (pp.46–48).

SPECIAL CASE
SUDDEN CARDIAC ARREST

If you see the casualty suddenly lose consciousness and fall to the ground, or other witnesses describe those symptoms, assume sudden cardiac arrest and immediately start CPR with chest compressions (pp.66–67).

THE ABC CHECK

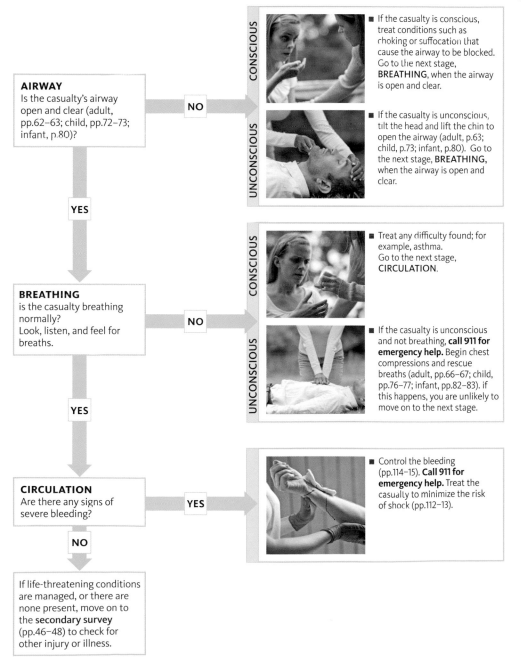

AIRWAY
Is the casualty's airway open and clear (adult, pp.62–63; child, pp.72–73; infant, p.80)?

NO — CONSCIOUS

- If the casualty is conscious, treat conditions such as choking or suffocation that cause the airway to be blocked. Go to the next stage, **BREATHING**, when the airway is open and clear.

UNCONSCIOUS

- If the casualty is unconscious, tilt the head and lift the chin to open the airway (adult, p.63; child, p.73; infant, p.80). Go to the next stage, **BREATHING**, when the airway is open and clear.

YES

BREATHING
is the casualty breathing normally?
Look, listen, and feel for breaths.

NO — CONSCIOUS

- Treat any difficulty found; for example, asthma. Go to the next stage, **CIRCULATION**.

UNCONSCIOUS

- If the casualty is unconscious and not breathing, **call 911 for emergency help.** Begin chest compressions and rescue breaths (adult, pp.66–67; child, pp.76–77; infant, pp.82–83). if this happens, you are unlikely to move on to the next stage.

YES

CIRCULATION
Are there any signs of severe bleeding?

YES

- Control the bleeding (pp.114–15). **Call 911 for emergency help.** Treat the casualty to minimize the risk of shock (pp.112–13).

NO

If life-threatening conditions are managed, or there are none present, move on to the **secondary survey** (pp.46–48) to check for other injury or illness.

SECONDARY SURVEY

Once you have completed the primary survey and dealt with any life-threatening conditions, start the methodical process of checking for other injuries or illnesses by performing a head-to-toe examination. This is called the secondary survey. Question the casualty and the people around him. Make a note of your findings if you can, and pass all the details to the emergency services or hospital, or whoever takes responsibility for the casualty (p.29).

Ideally, the casualty should remain in the position found, at least until you are satisfied that it is safe to move him into a more comfortable position appropriate for his injury or illness.

This survey includes two further checks beyond the ABC (pp.44–45).

- **Disability** is the casualty's level of response (p.52).
- **Examine the casualty.** You may need to remove or cut away clothing to examine and/or treat the injuries.

By conducting this survey you are aiming to discover the following:

- **History** What happened leading up to the injury or sudden illness and any relevant medical history.
- **Symptoms** Information that the casualty gives you about his condition.
- **Signs** you find on examination of the casualty.

HISTORY

There are two important aspects to the history: what happened, and any previous medical history.

EVENT HISTORY

The first consideration is to find out what happened. Your initial questions should help you discover the immediate events leading up to the incident. The casualty can usually tell you this, but sometimes you have to rely on information from people nearby so it is important to verify that they are telling you facts and not just their opinions. There may also be clues, such as the impact on a vehicle, which can indicate the likely nature of the casualty's injury. This is often referred to as the mechanism of injury (pp.42–43).

PREVIOUS MEDICAL HISTORY

The second aspect to consider is a person's medical history. While this may have nothing to do with the present condition, it could be a clue to the cause. Clues to the existence of such a condition may include a medical bracelet or medication in the casualty's possessions (p.48).

TAKING A HISTORY

- **Ask what happened;** for example, establish whether the incident is due to illness or an accident.
- **Ask about medication** the casualty is taking.
- **Ask about medical history.** Find out if there are ongoing and previous conditions.
- **Find out** if a person has any allergies, including to any medications or latex.
- **Check when** the person last had something to eat or drink.
- **Note the presence of a medical warning bracelet**—this may indicate an ongoing medical condition, such as epilepsy, diabetes, or anaphylaxis.

SYMPTOMS

These are the sensations that the casualty feels and describes to you. When you talk to the casualty, ask him to give you as much detail as possible. For example, if he complains of pain, ask where it is. Ask him to describe the pain (is it constant or intermittent, sharp or dull). Ask him what makes the pain better (or worse), whether it is affected by movement or breathing, and, if it did not result from an injury, where and how it began. The casualty may describe other symptoms, too, such as nausea, giddiness, heat, cold, or thirst. Listen very carefully to his answers (p.20) and do not interrupt him while he is speaking.

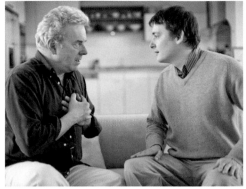

Listen to the casualty
Make eye contact with the casualty as you talk to him. Keep your questions simple, and listen carefully to the symptoms he describes.

SIGNS

These are features such as swelling, bleeding, discoloration, deformity, and smells that you can detect by observing and feeling the casualty, rather than asking the casualty questions. Use your senses—look, listen, feel, and smell—to get a complete picture. Always compare the injured and uninjured sides of the body. You may also notice that the person is unable to perform normal functions, such as moving his limbs or standing. Make a note of any obvious superficial injuries, going back to treat them only when you have completed your examination.

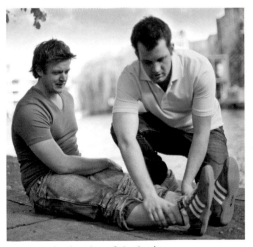

Compare both sides of the body
Always compare the injured part of the body with the uninjured side. Check for swelling, deformity, and discoloration.

QUICK REMINDER

Use the mnemonic **A M P L E** as a reminder when assessing a casualty to ensure that you have covered all aspects of the casualty's history. When the emergency services arrive, they may ask:
A—Allergy—does the person have any allergies?
M—Medications—is the person on any medication?
P—Previous medical history—do you know of any preexisting conditions?
L—Last meal—when did the person last eat?
E—Event history—what happened?

❮❮ SECONDARY SURVEY

LOOK FOR EXTERNAL CLUES

As part of your assessment, look for external clues to a casualty's condition. If you suspect drug abuse, take care because he may be carrying needles and syringes. You may find an appointment card for a hospital or clinic, or a card indicating a history of allergy, diabetes, or epilepsy. Horseback-riders or cyclists may carry such a card inside their riding hat or helmet. Food or medication may also give valuable clues about the casualty's condition; for example, people with diabetes may carry sugar packets or glucose gel. A person with a known disorder may have medical warning information on a special bracelet or medallion, (such as a "MedicAlert"). Keep any such item with the casualty or give it to the emergency services.

If you need to search a casualty's belongings, always try to ask first and perform the search in front of a reliable witness (p.21).

MEDICAL CLUES	
	MEDICATION A casualty may be carrying medication such as anti-inflammatories for back pain or nitroglycerine for angina.
	MEDICAL BRACELET This may be inscribed with information about a casualty's medical history (e.g., epilepsy, diabetes, or anaphylaxis), or there may be a number to call.
	PUFFER/INHALER The presence of an inhaler usually indicates that the casualty has asthma or other diseases that can cause wheezing or difficulty breathing.
	INSULIN PEN This may indicate that a person has diabetes. The casualty may also have a glucose testing kit.
	AUTO-INJECTOR This contains epinephrine (adrenaline), for people at risk of anaphylactic shock. The pens are color coded for adult and child doses.

HEAD-TO-TOE EXAMINATION

Once you have taken the casualty's history (p.46) and asked about any symptoms she has (p.47), you should carry out a detailed examination. Use your senses when you examine a casualty: look, listen, feel, and smell. Always start at the head and work down; this "head-to-toe" routine is both easily remembered and thorough. You may have to open, cut away, or remove clothing that is covering an injury, or if the casualty feels pain in a particular area. Always be sensitive to a casualty's privacy and dignity, and ask her permission before doing this.

Protect yourself and the casualty by wearing disposable gloves. Make sure that you do not move the casualty more than is strictly necessary. If possible, examine a conscious casualty in the position in which you find her, or one that best suits her condition, unless her life is in immediate danger. If an unconscious breathing casualty has been placed in the recovery position, leave her in this position while you carry out the head-to-toe examination.

Check the casualty's breathing and pulse rates (pp.52–53), then work from her head downward. Initially, note minor injuries but continue your examination to make sure that you do not miss any concealed potentially serious conditions; return to them only when you have completed your examination.

POSSIBLE FINDINGS ON CARRYING OUT AN EXAMINATION	
METHOD OF IDENTIFICATION	**SYMPTOMS OR SIGNS**
The casualty may tell you of these symptoms	■ Pain ■ Anxiety ■ Heat ■ Cold ■ Loss of sensation ■ Abnormal sensation ■ Thirst ■ Nausea ■ Tingling ■ Pain on touch or pressure ■ Faintness ■ Stiffness ■ Momentary unconsciousness ■ Weakness ■ Memory loss ■ Dizziness ■ Sensation of broken bone ■ Sense of impending doom
You may see these signs	■ Anxiety and painful expression ■ Unusual chest movement ■ Burns ■ Sweating ■ Wounds ■ Bleeding from orifices ■ Response to touch ■ Response to speech ■ Bruising ■ Abnormal skin color ■ Muscle spasm ■ Swelling ■ Deformity ■ Foreign bodies ■ Needle marks ■ Vomit ■ Incontinence ■ Loss of normal movement ■ Containers and other circumstantial evidence
You may feel these signs	■ Dampness ■ Abnormal body temperature ■ Swelling ■ Deformity ■ Irregularity ■ Grating bone ends
You may hear these signs	■ Noisy or distressed breathing ■ Groaning ■ Sucking sounds from a penetrating chest injury ■ Response to touch ■ Response to speech ■ Grating bone (crepitus)
You may smell these signs	■ Acetone ■ Alcohol ■ Burning ■ Gas or fumes ■ Solvents or glue ■ Urine ■ Feces ■ Cannabis

« HEAD-TO-TOE EXAMINATION

WHAT TO DO

1 Assess breathing (p.52). Check the rate (fast or slow), depth (shallow or deep), and nature (is it easy or difficult, noisy or quiet). Check the pulse (p.53). Assess the rate (fast or slow), rhythm (regular or irregular) and strength (strong or weak).

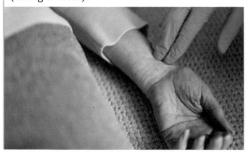

2 Start the physical examination at the casualty's head. Run your hands carefully over the scalp to feel for bleeding, swelling, or depression, which may indicate a fracture. Be careful not to move the casualty if you suspect that she may have injured her neck.

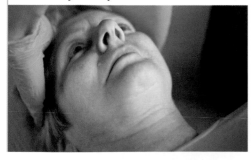

3 Speak clearly to the casualty in both ears to find out if she responds or if she can hear. Look for clear fluid or watery blood coming from either ear. These discharges may be signs of a serious head injury (pp.144–45).

4 Examine both eyes. Note whether they are open. Check the size of the pupils (the black area). If the pupils are not the same size it may indicate head injury. Look for any foreign object, or blood in the whites of the eyes.

5 Check the nose for discharges as you did for the ears. Look for clear fluid or watery blood (or a mixture of both) coming from either nostril. Soot around the nostrils or singed nasal hairs might indicate serious airway burns.

6 Look in the mouth for anything that might obstruct the airway. If the casualty has dentures that are intact and fit firmly, leave them. Look for mouth wounds or burns and check for irregularity in the line of the teeth.

7 Look at the skin. Note the color and temperature: is it pale, flushed, or gray-blue (cyanosis); is it hot or cold, dry or damp? Pale, cold, sweaty (clammy) skin suggests shock; a flushed, hot face suggests fever or heatstroke. A blue tinge indicates lack of oxygen; look for this in the lips, ears, and face.

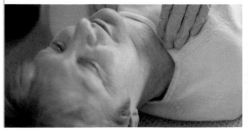

8 Loosen clothing around the neck, and look for signs such as a medical warning necklace (p.48) or a hole (stoma) in the windpipe. Run your fingers gently along the spine from the base of the skull down as far as possible without moving the casualty; check for irregularity, swelling, tenderness, or deformity.

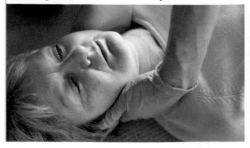

9 Look at the chest. Ask the casualty to breathe deeply, and note whether the chest expands evenly, easily, and equally on both sides. Feel the rib cage to check for deformity, irregularity, or tenderness. Ask the casualty if she is aware of grating sensations when breathing, and listen for unusual sounds. Note whether breathing causes any pain. Look for any external injuries, such as bleeding or stab wounds.

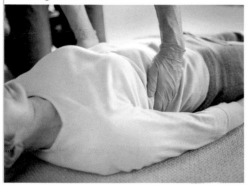

10 Feel along the collarbones, shoulders, upper arms, elbows, hands, and fingers for any swelling, tenderness, or deformity. Check the movements of the elbows, wrists, and fingers by asking the casualty to bend and straighten each joint.

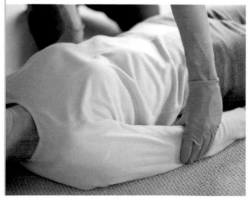

11 Check that the casualty has no abnormal sensations in the arms or fingers. If the fingertips are pale or gray-blue there may be a problem with blood circulation. Look out for needle marks on the forearms, or a medical warning bracelet (p.48).

12 If there is any impairment in movement or loss of sensation in the limbs, do not move the casualty to examine the spine, since these signs suggest spinal injury. Otherwise, gently pass your hand under the hollow of the back and check for swelling and tenderness.

13 Gently feel the casualty's abdomen to detect any evidence of bleeding, and to identify any rigidity or tenderness of the abdomen's muscular wall, which could be a sign of internal bleeding. Compare one side of the abdomen with the other. Note any bruising on the abdomen or pelvis.

14 Feel both sides of the hips, and examine the pelvis for signs of fracture. Check clothing for any evidence of incontinence, which suggests spinal or bladder injury, or bleeding from orifices, which suggests pelvic fracture.

15 Check the legs. Look and feel for bleeding, swelling, deformity, or tenderness. Ask the casualty to raise each leg in turn, and to move her ankles and knees.

16 Check the movement and feeling in the toes. Check that the vicitm has no abnormal sensations in her feet or toes. Compare the feet. Look at the skin color: gray-blue skin may indicate a circulatory disorder or an injury due to cold.

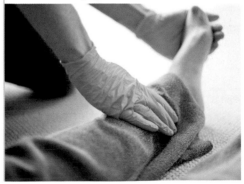

MONITORING VITAL SIGNS

When treating a casualty, you may need to assess and monitor his breathing, pulse, and level of response. This information can help you identify problems and indicate changes in a casualty's condition. Monitoring should be repeated regularly, and your findings recorded

and handed over to the medical assistance taking over (p.21).

In addition, if a casualty has a condition that affects his body temperature, such as fever, heatstroke, or hypothermia, you will also need to monitor his temperature.

LEVEL OF RESPONSE

You need to monitor a casualty's level of response to assess her level of consciousness and any change in her condition. Any injury or illness that affects the brain may affect consciousness, and any deterioration is potentially serious. Assess the level of response using the AVPU scale (right) and make a note of any deterioration or improvement.

- **A**—Is the casualty **Alert?** Are her eyes open and does she respond to questions?
- **V**—**Does the casualty respond to Voice?** Can she answer questions and obey commands?
- **P**—**Does the casualty respond to Pain?** Does she open her eyes or move if pinched?
- **U**—**Is the casualty Unresponsive** to any stimulus (i.e. unconscious)?

BREATHING

When assessing a casualty's breathing, check the breathing rate and listen for any breathing difficulties or unusual noises.

An adult's normal breathing rate is 12–16 breaths per minute; in babies and young children, it is 20–30 breaths per minute. When checking breathing, listen for breaths and watch the casualty's chest movements. For a baby or young child, it might be easier to place your hand on the chest and feel for movement of breathing. Record the following information:

- **Rate**—count the number of breaths per minute.
- **Depth**—are the breaths deep or shallow
- **Ease**—are the breaths easy, difficult or painful?
- **Noise**—is the breathing quiet or noisy, and if noisy, what are the types of noise?

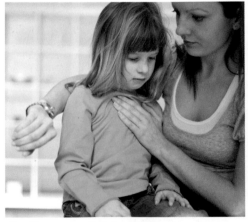

Checking a casualty's breathing rate
Observe the chest movements and count the number of breaths per minute. Use a watch to time breaths. For a baby or young child, place your hand on the chest and feel for movement.

PULSE

Each heartbeat creates a wave of pressure as blood is pumped along the arteries (pp.108–09). Where arteries lie close to the skin surface, such as on the inside of the wrist and at the neck, this pressure wave can be felt as a pulse. The normal pulse rate in adults is 60–100 beats per minute. The rate is faster in children and may be slower in very fit adults. An abnormally fast or slow pulse may be a sign of illness.

The pulse may be felt at the wrist (radial pulse), or if this is not possible, the neck (carotid pulse). In babies, the pulse in the upper arm (brachial pulse) is easier to find.

When checking a pulse, use your fingers (not your thumb) and press lightly against the skin. Record the following points.
- **Rate** (number of beats per minute).
- **Strength** (strong or weak).
- **Rhythm** (regular or irregular).

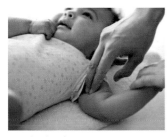

Brachial pulse
Place the pads of two fingers on the inner side of an infant's upper arm.

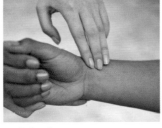

Radial pulse
Place the pads of two or three fingers below the wrist creases at the base of the thumb.

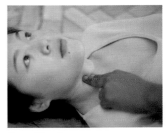

Carotid pulse
Place the pads of two fingers in the hollow between the large neck muscle and the windpipe.

BODY TEMPERATURE

Although not a vital sign, low or high body temperature may be an important indicator of a life-threatening problem. You can feel exposed skin but use a thermometer to obtain an accurate reading. Normal body temperature is 98.6°F (37°C) but can be slightly higher or lower. A temperature above 100.4°F (38°C) is usually caused by infection, but can be the result of heat exhaustion or heatstroke (pp.184–85). A lower body temperature may result from exposure to cold and/or wet conditions—hypothermia (p.186–88)—or it may be a sign of life-threatening infection or shock (pp.112–13). There are several different types of thermometer; see below.

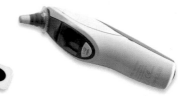

Digital thermometer
Used to measure temperature under the tongue or in the armpit. Leave it in place until it makes a beeping sound (about 30 seconds), then read the display.

Forehead thermometer
A heat-sensitive strip for use on a small child. Hold against the child's forehead for about 30 seconds. The color on the strip indicates temperature.

Ear sensor
Place the probe inside the ear. Press the measurement key wait for a beeping sound, then read the display. This thermometer can be used while a person is asleep.

4

To stay alive we need an adequate supply of oxygen to enter the lungs and be transferred to all cells in the body by the circulating blood. If a person is deprived of oxygen for any length of time, the brain will begin to fail. As a result, the casualty will eventually lose consciousness, breathing will cease, the heart will stop, and death results. The airway must be kept open so that breathing can occur, allowing oxygen to enter the lungs and be circulated in the body.

The priority of a first aider when treating any unconscious casualty is to assess for breathing and immediately begin CPR with chest compressions if breathing is absent. An automated external defibrillator (AED) may be required to "shock" the heart back into a normal rhythm. This chapter outlines the priorities to remember when dealing with a casualty who has lost consciousness for any reason.

There are important differences in the treatment of unconscious children and adults; this chapter gives separate step-by-step instructions for dealing with each of these groups.

AIMS AND OBJECTIVES

- To maintain an open airway, to check breathing and resuscitate if required.
- To **call 911 for emergency help.**

THE UNCONSCIOUS
CASUALTY

BREATHING AND CIRCULATION

Oxygen is essential to support life. Without it, cells in the body die—those in the brain survive only a few minutes without oxygen. Oxygen is taken in when we inhale (pp.90–91), and it is then circulated to all the body tissues via the circulatory system (p.108). It is vital to maintain breathing and circulation in order to sustain life.

The process of breathing enables air, which contains oxygen, to be taken into the air sacs (alveoli) in the lungs. Here, the oxygen is transferred across blood vessel walls into the blood, where it combines with blood cells. At the same time, the waste product of breathing,

carbon dioxide, is released and exhaled in the breath. When oxygen has been transferred to the blood cells it is carried from the lungs to the heart through the pulmonary veins. The heart pumps the oxygenated blood to the rest of the body via blood vessels called arteries.

After oxygen is given up to the body tissues, deoxygenated blood is brought back to the heart by blood vessels called veins (p.108). The heart pumps this blood to the lungs via the pulmonary arteries, where the carbon dioxide is released and the blood is reoxygenated before circulating around the body again.

Lungs

Fresh oxygen is drawn into the lungs via the nose and mouth by the windpipe (trachea)

Deoxygenated blood is pumped to the lungs by the heart through the pulmonary arteries

Oxygenated blood returns from the lungs to the heart

Oxygenated blood leaves the heart to be circulated around the body via the aorta

Deoxygenated blood returns from body tissue to the heart

Heart pumps oxygenated blood around the body

Red blood cell

Direction of oxygen flow

Air sac (alveolus)

Direction of carbon dioxide flow

How the heart and lungs work together

Air containing oxygen is taken into the lungs via the mouth and nose. Blood is pumped from the heart to the lungs, where it absorbs oxygen. Oxygenated blood is returned to the heart before being pumped around the body.

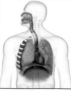

Exchange of gases in the air sacs

Carbon dioxide passes out of blood cells into air sacs (alveoli). Oxygen crosses the walls of alveoli into blood cells.

LIFE-SAVING PRIORITIES

The procedures set out in this chapter can maintain a casualty's circulation and breathing until emergency help arrives.

With an unconscious casualty who is not breathing normally, your priorities can be remembered by the initials C-A-B. Upon determining that the casualty is not breathing, begin chest compressions (C) immediately to maintain blood circulation (to get oxygenated blood to the tissues). After providing the initial circulation for the casualty, it is important to maintain an open airway (A) and to breathe for the casualty (B) to get oxygen into the body. In an adult during the first minutes after the heart stops (cardiac arrest), the blood oxygen level remains constant, so chest compressions are more important than rescue breaths in the initial phase of resuscitation. After two to four minutes, the blood oxygen level falls and rescue breathing becomes important as well. The combination of chest compressions and rescue breaths is called cardiopulmonary resuscitation, or CPR. In a child or infant, a problem with breathing is the most likely reason for the heart to stop.

In addition to CPR, a machine called an automated external defibrillator (AED) can be used to deliver an electric shock that may restore a normal heartbeat (pp.84–87).

CHEST COMPRESSION–ONLY CPR

If you have not had any formal training in CPR, or you are unwilling or unable to give rescue breaths, you can give chest compressions only. The 911 dispatcher will give instructions for performing chest compression-only CPR (pp.70–71).

EARLY HELP **Call 911 for emergency help.** Look for an available AED or send a bystander for one.	**EARLY CPR** Chest compressions and rescue breaths are used to "buy time" until expert help arrives.	**EARLY DEFIBRILLATION** A controlled electric shock from an AED is given. This can "shock" the heart into a normal rhythm.	**EARLY ADVANCED CARE** Specialized treatment by paramedics and in the hospital stabilizes the casualty's condition.

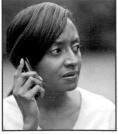 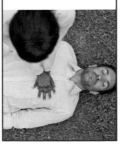 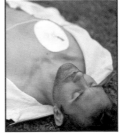 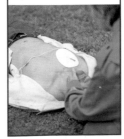

Chain of survival
Four elements increase the chances of a collapsed casualty surviving. If any one of the elements in this chain is missing, the chances of survival are reduced.

« LIFE-SAVING PRIORITIES

IMPORTANCE OF MAINTAINING CIRCULATION

If the heart stops beating, blood does not circulate through the body. As a result, vital organs—most importantly the brain—become starved of oxygen. Brain cells are unable to survive for more than three to four minutes without a supply of oxygen.

Some circulation can be maintained artificially by chest compressions (pp.66–67). These act as a mechanical aid to the heart in order to get blood flowing around the body. Pushing vertically down on the center of the chest increases the pressure in the chest cavity, expelling blood from the heart and forcing it into the tissues. As pressure on the chest is released, the chest recoils, or comes back up, and more blood is "sucked" into the heart; this blood is then forced out of the heart by the next compression.

To ensure that the blood is supplied with enough oxygen, chest compressions should be combined with rescue breathing (opposite). However, even if you do not feel comfortable providing rescue breaths or are not trained to do so, it is very important that you still provide chest compressions.

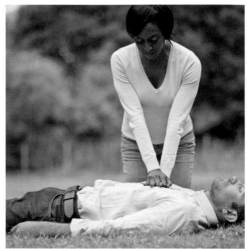

GIVING CHEST COMPRESSIONS

RESTORING HEART RHYTHM

A machine called an AED (automated external defibrillator) can be used to attempt to restart the heart when it has stopped (pp.84–87). The earlier the AED is used, the greater the chance of the casualty surviving. With each minute's delay, the casualty's chances of survival fall. AEDs can be used safely and effectively without training.

These machines can now be found in many public places, such as railroad and bus stations, shopping centers, airports, and government buildings. They are generally housed in cabinets, often marked with a lightning bolt, and placed where they can be easily found and accessed. The cabinets are not locked, but most are fitted with an alarm that is activated when the door is opened.

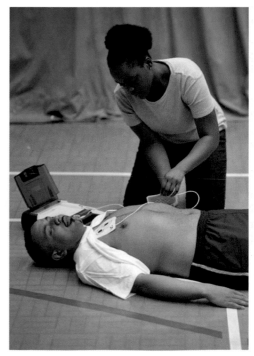

USING AN AUTOMATED EXTERNAL DEFIBRILLATOR

AN OPEN AIRWAY

An unconscious casualty's airway can become narrowed or blocked. This may be due to muscular control being lost, which allows the tongue to fall back and block the airway. When this happens, the casualty's breathing becomes difficult and noisy and may stop. Lifting the chin and tilting the head back lifts the tongue away from the entrance to the air passage, allowing delivery of rescue breaths.

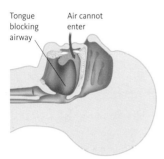

Tongue blocking airway

Air cannot enter

Blocked airway
In an unconscious casualty, the tongue falls back, blocking the throat and airway.

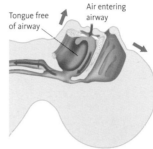

Tongue free of airway

Air entering airway

Open airway
In the head tilt, chin lift position, the tongue is lifted from the back of the throat and the trachea is open, so the airway will be clear.

BREATHING FOR A CASUALTY

Exhaled air contains about 16 percent oxygen (only five percent less than inhaled air) and a small amount of carbon dioxide. Your exhaled breath therefore contains enough oxygen to supply another person with oxygen—and potentially keep him alive—when it is forced into his lungs during rescue breathing.

By giving rescue breaths (p.67), you force air into his air passages. This reaches the air sacs (alveoli) in the lungs, and oxygen is then transferred through tiny blood vessels (capillaries) to red blood cells.

When you take your mouth away from the casualty's, his chest falls, and air containing waste products is pushed out, or exhaled, from his lungs. This process, performed together with chest compressions (pp.66–67), can supply the tissues with oxygen until help arrives.

> **CAUTION**
>
> AGONAL BREATHING
> This type of breathing usually takes the form of short, irregular gasps for breath. It is common in the first few minutes after a cardiac arrest. It should not be mistaken for normal breathing and, if it is present, chest compressions and rescue breaths (cardiopulmonary resuscitation/CPR) should be started without hesitation.

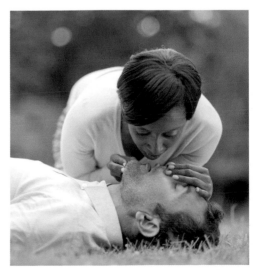

GIVING RESCUE BREATHS

« LIFE-SAVING PRIORITIES

ADULT RESUSCITATION

This action plan shows the order for the techniques you need to use when attending a collapsed adult. The plan assumes that you have already established that neither you nor the casualty is in immediate danger. More detailed explanations of each of the techniques shown here are given on the following pages.

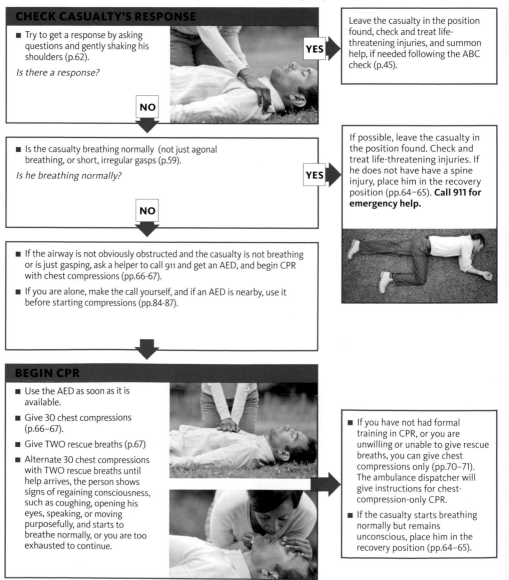

CHECK CASUALTY'S RESPONSE

- Try to get a response by asking questions and gently shaking his shoulders (p.62).

Is there a response?

YES

Leave the casualty in the position found, check and treat life-threatening injuries, and summon help, if needed following the ABC check (p.45).

NO

- Is the casualty breathing normally (not just agonal breathing, or short, irregular gasps (p.59).

Is he breathing normally?

YES

If possible, leave the casualty in the position found. Check and treat life-threatening injuries. If he does not have have a spine injury, place him in the recovery position (pp.64–65). **Call 911 for emergency help.**

NO

- If the airway is not obviously obstructed and the casualty is not breathing or is just gasping, ask a helper to call 911 and get an AED, and begin CPR with chest compressions (pp.66-67).
- If you are alone, make the call yourself, and if an AED is nearby, use it before starting compressions (pp.84-87).

BEGIN CPR

- Use the AED as soon as it is available.
- Give 30 chest compressions (p.66–67).
- Give TWO rescue breaths (p.67)
- Alternate 30 chest compressions with TWO rescue breaths until help arrives, the person shows signs of regaining consciousness, such as coughing, opening his eyes, speaking, or moving purposefully, and starts to breathe normally, or you are too exhausted to continue.

- If you have not had formal training in CPR, or you are unwilling or unable to give rescue breaths, you can give chest compressions only (pp.70–71). The ambulance dispatcher will give instructions for chest-compression-only CPR.
- If the casualty starts breathing normally but remains unconscious, place him in the recovery position (pp.64–65).

CHILD/INFANT RESUSCITATION

This action plan shows the order for the techniques to use when attending a child between the ages of one and puberty or an infant under one year. A breathing problem is the most likely cause of cardiac arrest but chest compressions are given first.

CHECK CHILD'S RESPONSE

- Try to get a response by asking questions and gently tapping the child's shoulder or an infant's foot.

Is there a response?

 NO

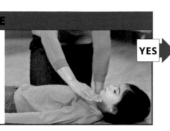

YES ▶

Leave the child in the position found, Use the primary survey (pp.44–45) to identify the serious injury and treat in order of priority.

Is she breathing normally?

NO

YES ▶

If possible, leave the casualty in the position found. Check and treat life-threatening injuries. If she does not have have a spine injury, place the child in the recovery position (pp.74–75), or hold infant (p.81). **Call 911 for emergency help.**

Send a helper to **call 911 for emergency help.**
- Ask the helper to bring an AED, preferably one with pediatric pads (pp.84–87). For an infant (under 1 year of age), a manual external defribrillator is preferred, but if it is not available, an adult AED can be used.
- If you are alone, perform 2 minutes of CPR, beginning with chest compressions, and then call 911, and if an AED is nearby, use it.

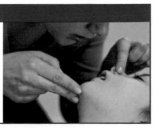

BEGIN CPR

- Give 30 chest compressions (child, p.76, or infant, p.83).
- Follow with 2 rescue breaths.
- Allternate 30 chest compressions with 2 rescue breaths until emergency help arrives, the child starts breathing normally or you are too exhausted to continue.

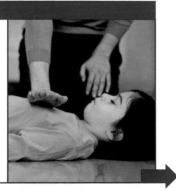

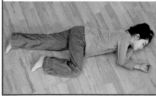

- It is better to give a combination of rescue breaths and chest compressions with infants and children. However, if you have not had formal training in CPR, or you are unwilling or unable to give rescue breaths, you may give chest compressions only (pp.70–71). The dispatcher will give instructions for chest-compression-only CPR.

- If the child starts breathing normally but remains unconscious, place her in the recovery position (child, pp.74–75, infant, p.81).

GIVING RESCUE BREATHS

- Tilt the head back and lift the chin to open the airway (child, p.77, or infant, p.83).
- Carefully remove any visible obstruction from the mouth.
- Give TWO rescue breaths.

UNCONSCIOUS ADULT

The following pages describe techniques for the management of an unconscious adult who may require resuscitation.

Always approach and treat the casualty from the side, kneeling down next to his head or chest. You will then be in the correct position to perform all stages of resuscitation: checking responsiveness and breathing; chest compressions; opening the airway; and giving rescue breaths (together called cardiopulmonary resuscitation, or CPR). At each stage in the process you will have decisions to make—for example, is the casualty breathing? The steps given here tell you what to do next.

The first priority is to determine responsiveness and to assess breathing. If the casualty is not responsive and not breathing or just gasping, you must begin chest compressions. If the casualty is breathing, place him in the recovery position. If you find the casualty slumped or not on his back, and you do not suspect a spinal injury, first place him on his back so that you can best assess him.

CAUTION
■ Always assume that there is a neck injury and shake the shoulders very gently.

HOW TO CHECK RESPONSE

On discovering a collapsed casualty, you should first make sure the scene is safe and then establish whether he is conscious or unconscious. Do this by gently shaking the casualty's shoulders. Ask "What happened?" or give a command such as, "Open your eyes." Always speak loudly and clearly to the casualty.

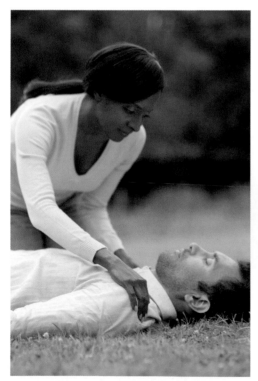

IF THERE IS A RESPONSE

1 **If there is no further danger,** leave the casualty in the position in which he was found, check for life-threatening injuries, and summon help if needed.

2 **Treat any condition found and monitor and record vital signs**—level of response, breathing, and pulse (pp.52–53)—until emergency help arrives or the casualty recovers.

IF THERE IS NO RESPONSE

1 **Shout for help.** Leave the casualty in the position in which he was found and assess for breathing.

2 **If you are unable to assess** the casualty for breathing in the position in which he was found, get help to turn him over using the log-roll technique (p.159). If seeking help to roll the casualty will cause significant delay, you should roll him yourself, as carefully as possible.

HOW TO CHECK BREATHING

In an unresponsive casualty, simply look at him to see whether or not he is breathing normally. Occasional gasps (agonal breathing) do not constitute normal breathing, and if you see this, you should treat it as if he were not breathing at all and begin chest compressions.

IF THE CASUALTY IS NOT BREATHING

 Send a helper to **call 911 for emergency help.** Ask the person to bring an AED if one is available. If you are alone, make the call yourself unless the condition is the result of drowning (p.100).

 Begin CPR with chest compressions (pp.66–67).

IF THE CASUALTY IS BREATHING

 Check the casualty for any life-threatening injuries, such as severe bleeding, and treat as necessary.

 Place the casualty in the recovery position (pp.64–65) and **call 911 for emergency help.**

 Monitor and record vital signs—level of response, breathing and pulse (pp.52–53) —while waiting for help to arrive.

« UNCONSCIOUS ADULT

HOW TO PLACE CASUALTY IN RECOVERY POSITION

If the casualty is found lying on his side or front, rather than his back, not all the following steps will be necessary to place him in the recovery position. If the mechanisms of injury suggest a spinal injury, treat as on pp.157–59.

WHAT TO DO

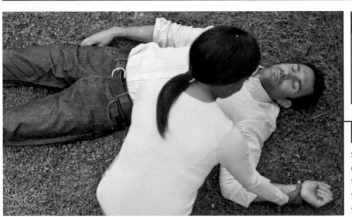

1 **Kneel beside the casualty.** Remove his glasses and any bulky objects, such as mobile phones or large bunches of keys, from his pockets. Do not search his pockets for small items.

2 **Make sure that both** of the casualty's legs are straight. Place the arm that is closest to you at right angles to the casualty's body, with the elbow bent and the palm facing upward.

3 **Bring the arm that is** farthest from you across the casualty's chest, and hold the back of his hand against the cheek closest to you. With your other hand, grasp the far leg just above the knee and pull it up, keeping the foot flat on the ground.

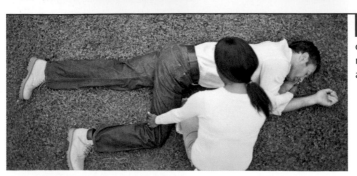

4 **Keeping the casualty's** hand pressed against his cheek, pull on the far leg and roll the casualty toward you and onto his side.

5 **Adjust the upper leg** so that both the hip and the knee are bent at right angles.

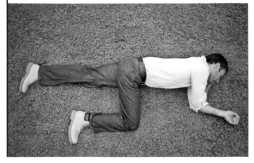

6 **Tilt the casualty's head back** and tilt his chin so that the airway remains open (p.63).

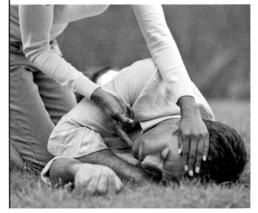

7 **If necessary, adjust the hand** under the cheek to keep the airway open.

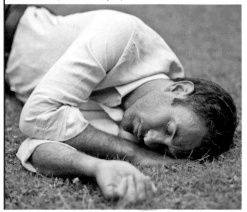

8 **If it has not already** been done, **call 911 for emergency help.** Monitor and record vital signs—level of response, breathing, and pulse (pp.52–53)—while waiting for help to arrive.

9 **If the casualty has to be left** in the recovery position for longer than 30 minutes, roll him onto his back, and then roll him onto the opposite side—unless other injuries prevent you from doing this.

SPECIAL CASE RECOVERY POSITION FOR SUSPECTED SPINAL INJURY

If you suspect a spinal injury (pp.157–59) and need to place the casualty in the recovery position, try to keep the spine straight.

- If you are alone, use the technique shown opposite and above.
- If you have a helper, one of you should steady the head while the other turns the casualty (right).
- With three people, one person should steady the head while another turns the casualty. The third person should keep the casualty's back straight during the maneuver.
- If there are four or more people in total, use the log-roll technique (p.159).

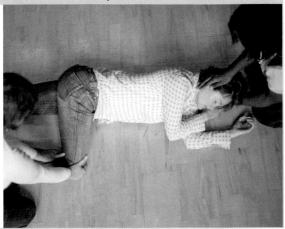

« UNCONSCIOUS ADULT

HOW TO GIVE CPR

WHAT TO DO

1 **Kneel beside the casualty** level with his chest. Place the heel of one hand on the center of the casualty's chest. You can identify the correct hand position for chest compressions through a casualty's clothing.

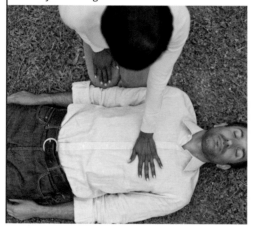

HAND POSITION

Place your hand on the casualty's breastbone as indicated here. Make sure that you do not press on the casualty's ribs, the lower tip of the breastbone (the xiphoid process), or the upper abdomen.

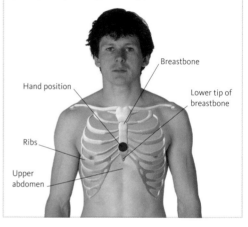

Breastbone

Hand position

Lower tip of breastbone

Ribs

Upper abdomen

2 **Place the heel of your other hand** on top of the first hand, and interlock your fingers, making sure the fingers are kept off the ribs.

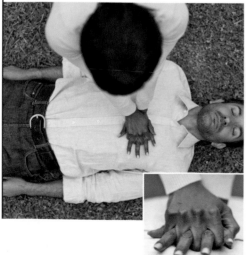

3 **Leaning over the casualty,** with your arms straight, press down vertically on the breastbone and depress the chest by at least 2 in (5 cm). Release the pressure without removing your hands from his chest. Allow the chest to come back up fully (recoil) before giving the next compression.

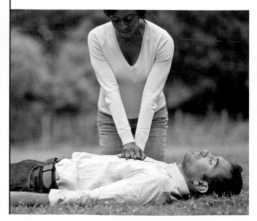

4 **Compress the chest** 30 times at a rate of at least 100 compressions per minute. The time taken for compression and release should be about the same.

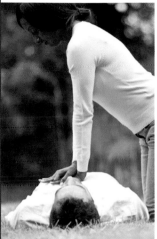

5 **Open the airway** with the head tilt–chin lift maneuver: put one hand on his forehead and two fingers of the other hand under the bony tip of his chin. Move the hand that was on the forehead down to pinch the soft part of the nose with the finger and thumb. Allow the casualty's mouth to fall open.

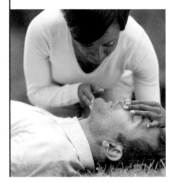

CAUTION

If there is more than one rescuer, change over every 2 minutes (after 5 cycles of CPR) with minimal interruption to chest compressions.

6 **Take a breath** and place your lips around the casualty's mouth, making sure you have a good seal. Blow into the casualty's mouth until his chest rises. A complete rescue breath should take one second. If the chest does not rise, you may need to adjust the head position (p.63).

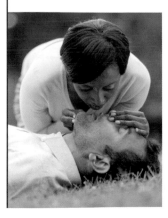

7 **Maintaining head tilt** and chin lift, take your mouth off the casualty's mouth and look to see his chest fall. If his chest rises visibly as you blow and falls fully when you lift your mouth away, you have given a rescue breath. Give a second rescue breath.

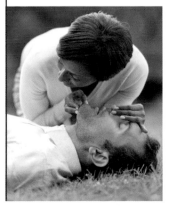

8 **Continue the cycle** of 30 chest compressions followed by 2 rescue breaths until: emergency help arrives and takes over; the casualty shows signs of regaining consciousness, such as coughing, opening his eyes, moving purposefully, and starts to breathe normally; or you are too exhausted to continue.

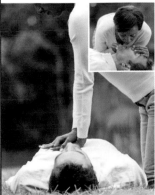

« UNCONSCIOUS ADULT

SPECIAL CONSIDERATIONS FOR CPR

There are circumstances that make the normal steps for CPR more challenging. For example:

- If you have not been trained in CPR or are unwilling or unable to give rescue breaths, you can give chest compressions only (pp.70–71). If you call 911, the dispatcher will give you instructions for compression-only CPR.
- If there is more than one rescuer, change over every 2 minutes, with minimal interruption to chest compressions.
- If the casualty vomits during CPR, roll him away from you onto his side, ensuring that his head is turned toward the floor to allow vomit to drain away. Clear any residual debris from his mouth, then immediately roll him onto his back again and recommence CPR.
- If a woman in the late stages of pregnancy requires CPR, raise her right hip off the ground by tilting it upward before you begin chest compressions (see below).
- Modified rescue breathing may be necessary in some cases: for example, if a casualty has mouth or oral injuries, you can give rescue breaths through the nose (opposite). A casualty may breathe through a hole in the front of the neck—a stoma (opposite). You can also use a pocket mask or face shield when giving rescue breaths.

CPR IN LATE STAGES OF PREGNANCY

If a heavily pregnant woman is lying on her back, the pregnant uterus will press against the large blood vessels in the abdomen. This restricts blood from the lower part of the body from returning to the heart, which reduces the amount of blood circulation that can be achieved with chest compressions. To prevent this from happening, tilt her right hip upward.

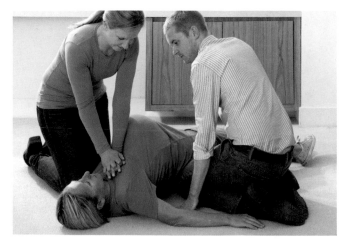

Positioning the woman
Keep the woman's upper body as flat on the floor as possible in order to give good-quality compressions. Raise her right hip and ask a helper to kneel beside the woman so that his knees are underneath the raised hip. If you are on your own, place tightly rolled up clothing or towels under the woman's hip to lift it.

PROBLEMS WITH RESCUE BREATHING

If a casualty's chest does not rise when giving rescue breaths:

- Recheck the head tilt and chin lift;
- Recheck the casualty's mouth. Remove any obvious obstructions, but do not do a finger sweep of the mouth.

Make no more than two attempts to achieve rescue breaths before repeating chest compressions.

VARIATIONS FOR RESCUE BREATHING

There are some cases where mouth-to-mouth rescue breaths are not appropriate and you need to use a mouth-to-nose or mouth-to-stoma technique.

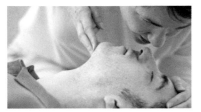

Mouth-to-nose rescue breathing
If a casualty has been rescued from the water, or injuries to the mouth make it impossible to achieve a good seal, you can use the mouth to-nose method for giving rescue breaths. With the casualty's mouth closed, form a tight seal with your lips around the casualty's nose and blow steadily into his nose. Then allow the mouth to fall open to let the air escape.

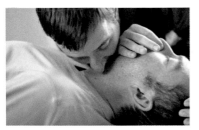

Mouth-to-stoma rescue breathing
A casualty who has had his voice box surgically removed breathes through an opening in the front of the neck (a stoma), rather than through the mouth and nose. Always check for a stoma before giving rescue breaths. If you find a stoma, close off the mouth and nose with one hand and then breathe into the stoma.

FACE SHIELDS AND POCKET MASKS
Face shields are plastic barriers with a filter that is placed over the casualty's mouth. A pocket mask has a mouthpiece through which breaths are given. If you know how to use one of these aids, you should carry it with you and use it whenever you need to resuscitate a casualty.

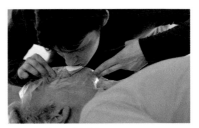

Using a face shield
Tilt the casualty's head back to open the airway. Place the shield over his face so the filter is over the mouth. Make a seal over the entire mouth area, and give rescue breaths through the filter.

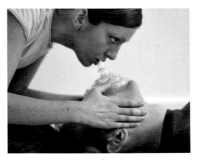

Using a pocket mask
Kneel behind the casualty's head. Open the airway and place the mask, narrow end toward you, over the casualty's mouth and nose. Deliver rescue breaths through the mouthpiece.

WHEN THE AMBULANCE ARRIVES

Tell the EMS personnel that you are a first aider and give a full report of what has happened. However, do not stop CPR while you are doing this unless they tell you to do so. Listen carefully to what they ask you to do and follow their instructions (p.23). If you have access to an AED (pp.84–87) and are trained to use it, you may have already attached it to the casualty's chest. If not, the EMS personnel will have one and attach it. You may be asked to continue with chest compressions while they do this. You will be asked to stand clear while it analyzes the casualty's heart rhythm (p.84). Do not approach the casualty again until asked to do so.

« UNCONSCIOUS ADULT

- If there is more than one rescuer swap every 2 minutes to prevent fatigue. Make sure there is minimal interruption when you change over to maintain the quality of the compressions.

- For unconscious children and babies who are not breathing, it is best to give CPR using rescue breaths with chest compressions (pp.76–77 and pp.82–83).

- If a casualty has been rescued from water and is not breathing, it is best to give CPR using rescue breaths and chest compressions (p.100).

CHEST-COMPRESSION-ONLY CPR

Healthcare professionals and trained first aiders will deliver CPR using chest compressions combined with rescue breaths (pp.66–67). However, if you have not been trained in CPR or you are unwilling or unable to give rescue breaths, chest-compression-only CPR has been shown to be of great benefit certainly in the first minutes after the heart has stopped. The dispatcher will give instructions for chest-compression-only resuscitation for a collapsed casualty when advising an untrained person by telephone. It is important to start chest compressions as soon as possible. You should give good-quality compressions and continue with them until emergency help arrives and takes over, or the casualty shows signs of regaining consciousness such as coughing, opening his eyes, speaking or moving purposefully and starts breathing normally, or you are too exhausted to continue.

WHAT TO DO

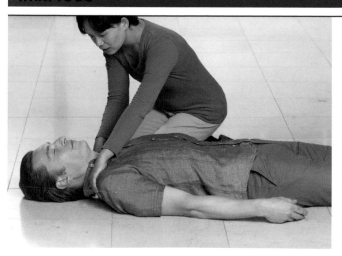

1 Check for a response.
Gently shake the casualty's shoulders, and talk to him or give a command (p.62).

IF THERE IS A RESPONSE
Use the primary survey (pp.44–45) to identify the most serious injury and treat conditions in order of priority.

IF THERE IS NO RESPONSE
Tell a helper to **call 911 for emergency help** and to get an AED. If you are alone, make the call yourself, and if an AED is nearby, retrieve and use it (pp.84–86).

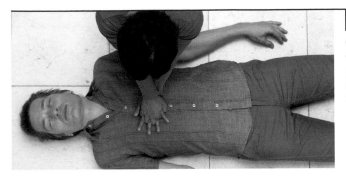

2 **Kneel beside the casualty,** level with his chest. Place one hand on the center of the chest (p.66)—you can identify the position through clothing. Put the heel of your other hand on top of the first and interlock your fingers.

3 **Begin chest compressions:** lean over the casualty, with your arms straight and press down vertically on his breastbone, depressing the chest by at least 2 in (5 cm). Release the pressure— but do not take your hands off the chest—and let the chest come back up. The time taken for compression and release should be about the same.

4 **Continue with compressions** at a rate of at least 100 per minute until emergency help arrives and takes over, or the casualty shows signs of regaining consciousness such as coughing, opening his eyes, speaking or moving purposefully and starts breathing normally, or you are too exhausted to continue.

> **CAUTION**
>
> ■ After 2 minutes of compression-only CPR, the body does need oxygen, so compressions should be combined with rescue breathing (pp.66–69).

UNCONSCIOUS CHILD (ONE YEAR TO PUBERTY)

The following pages describe the techniques that may be needed for the resuscitation of an unconscious child aged between one year and puberty.

When treating a child, always approach and treat her from the side, kneeling down next to the head or chest. You will then be in the correct position to carry out all the different stages of resuscitation: checking responsiveness and breathing; chest compressions; opening the airway; and giving rescue breaths (together called cardiopulmonary resuscitation, or CPR).

At each stage you will have decisions to make; for example, is the child breathing? The steps given here tell you what to do next. The first priority is to determine responsiveness and to assess breathing. If the casualty is not responsive and not breathing or just gasping, you must begin chest compressions. If the casualty is breathing, place in the recovery position (pp.74–75).

If a child with a known heart condition collapses, **call 911 for emergency help** immediately and ask for an AED to be brought (pp.84–87). Early access to advanced care can be life-saving.

HOW TO CHECK RESPONSE

On discovering a collapsed child, you should first establish whether she is conscious or unconscious. Do this by speaking loudly and clearly to the child. Ask "What happened?" or give a command such as, "Open your eyes." Place one hand on her shoulder, and gently tap her to see if there is a response.

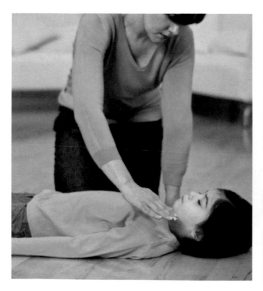

IF THERE IS A RESPONSE

 If there is no further danger, leave the child in the position in which she was found; check for life-threatening injuries and summon emergency help if needed.

Treat any condition found. Monitor and record vital signs—level of response, breathing, and pulse (pp.52–53)—until emergency help arrives or the child recovers.

IF THERE IS NO RESPONSE

Shout for help. Leave the child in the position in which she was found, and assess for breathing.

If you are unable to assess for breathing in the position in which she was found, roll the child onto her back using the log-roll technique (p.159).

HOW TO ASSESS BREATHING

In an unresponsive casualty, simply look at her to see whether or not she is breathing normally. Occasional gasps (agonal breathing) do not constitute normal breathing, and if you see this, you should treat it as if she were not breathing at all and begin chest compressions.

IF THE CHILD IS BREATHING

 Check for life-threatening injuries such as severe bleeding. Treat as necessary.

 Place the child in the recovery position (pp.74–75) and **call 911 for emergency help.**

 Monitor and record vital signs—level of response, breathing, and pulse (pp.52–53)—while waiting for help to arrive.

IF THE CHILD IS NOT BREATHING

 Ask a helper to **call 911 for emergency help** and to retrieve an AED if one is available, while you begin CPR with chest compressions (pp.76–77).

 If you are alone, perform chest compressions for 2 minutes and then **call 911 for emergency help** yourself. Continue with CPR, alternating cycles of 30 compressions with TWO breaths, until help arrives.

≪ UNCONSCIOUS CHILD

HOW TO PLACE CHILD IN RECOVERY POSITION

If the child is found lying on her side or front, rather than her back, not all of these steps will be necessary to place her in the recovery position. If the mechanisms of injury suggest a spinal injury, treat as on pp.157–59.

WHAT TO DO

1 Kneel beside the child. Remove her glasses and any bulky objects from her pockets, but do not search pockets for small items.

2 Make sure that both of the child's legs are straight. Place the arm nearest to you at right angles to the child's body, with the elbow bent and the palm facing upward.

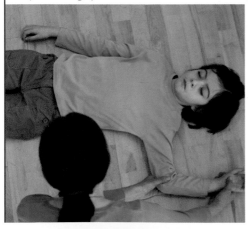

3 Bring the arm that is farthest from you across the child's chest, and hold the back of her hand against the cheek nearest to you. With your other hand, grasp the far leg just above the knee and pull it up, keeping the foot flat on the ground.

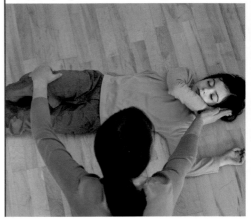

4 Keeping the child's hand pressed against her cheek, pull on the far leg and roll the child toward you and onto her side.

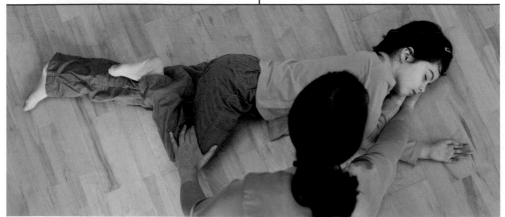

5 Adjust the upper leg so that both the hip and the knee are bent at right angles. Tilt the child's head back and lift the chin so that the airway remains open.

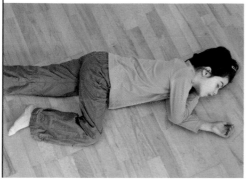

6 If necessary, adjust the hand under the cheek to make sure that the head remains tilted and the airway stays open. If it has not already been done, **call 911 for emergency help.** Monitor and record vital signs—level of response, breathing, and pulse (pp.52–53)—until help arrives.

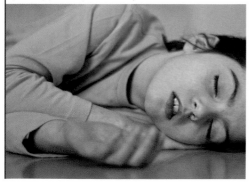

7 If the child has to be left in the recovery position for longer than 30 minutes, you should roll her onto her back, then turn her onto the opposite side—unless other injuries prevent you from doing this.

SPECIAL CASE RECOVERY POSITION FOR SUSPECTED SPINAL INJURY

If you suspect a spinal injury (pp.157–59) and need to place her in the recovery position, try to keep the spine straight using the following guidelines:

- If you are alone, use the technique shown below.
- If there are two of you, one person should steady the head while the other turns the child.
- If there are three of you, one person should steady the head while one person turns the child. The third person should keep the child's back straight during the maneuver.
- If there are four or more people in total, use the log-roll technique (p.159).

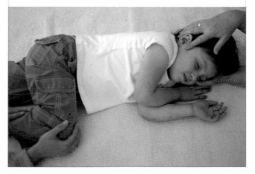

❰❰ UNCONSCIOUS CHILD

HOW TO GIVE CPR

WHAT TO DO

1 Determine unresponsiveness and assess breathing (not just gasping).

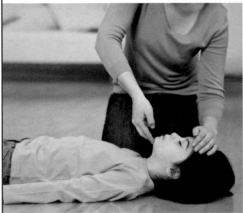

2 Kneel level with the child's chest. Place one hand on the center of her chest. This is the point at which you will apply pressure.

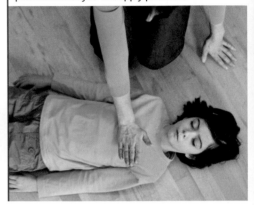

3 Lean over the child, with your arm straight, and then press down vertically on the breastbone with the heel of your hand. Depress the chest by at least one-third of its depth—about 2 in (5 cm). Release the pressure without removing your hand. Allow the chest to come back up completely (recoil) before you give the next compression. Compress the chest 30 times, at a rate of at least 100 compressions per minute. The time taken for compression and release should be about the same.

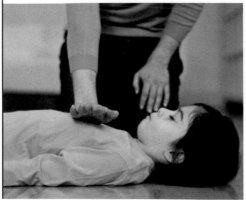

4 Open and assess the airway. Pick out any visible obstructions from the mouth. Do not sweep the mouth with your finger to look for obstructions.

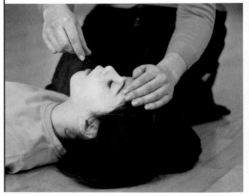

5 Pinch the soft part of the child's nose with the finger and thumb of the hand that was on the forehead. Make sure that her nostrils are closed to prevent air from escaping. Allow her mouth to fall open.

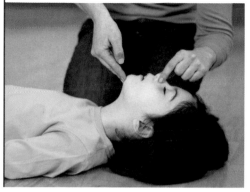

6 Take a deep breath in before placing your lips around the child's mouth, making sure that you form an airtight seal. Blow steadily into the child's mouth for one second; the chest should rise.

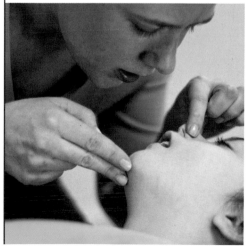

8 If you are alone, perform chest-compression-only CPR or CPR using cycles of **30** compressions followed by TWO rescue breaths, for two minutes, then stop to **call 911 for emergency help.** Continue CPR until emergency help takes over, the child starts to breathe normally, or you become too exhausted to continue.

CAUTION

If there are two rescuers, one should immediately call 911 while the other begins CPR. They can switch every two minutes.

HAND POSITION

Place one hand on the child's breastbone as indicated here. Make sure that you do not apply pressure over the child's ribs, the lower tip of the breastbone (the xiphoid process) or the upper abdomen.

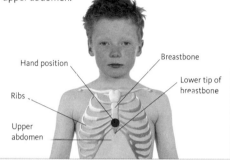

Hand position

Ribs

Upper abdomen

Breastbone

Lower tip of breastbone

7 Maintaining head tilt and chin lift, take your mouth off the child's mouth and look to see the chest fall. If the chest rises visibly as you blow and falls fully when you lift your mouth, you have given a rescue breath. If the chest does not rise you may need to adjust the head (p.78). Give TWO rescue breaths.

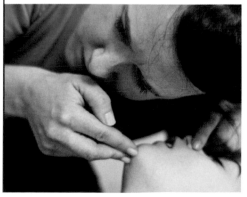

« UNCONSCIOUS CHILD ONE YEAR TO PUBERTY

SPECIAL CONSIDERATIONS FOR CPR

There are circumstances when it may be difficult to deliver CPR. While it is better to give a combination of rescue breaths and chest compressions, you may not have been formally trained in CPR or you may be unwilling or unable to give rescue breaths. In this situation you can give chest compressions only. When you call 911, the dispatcher will give instructions for chest-compression only CPR.

■ **If there is more than one rescuer,** change over every 2 minutes, with minimal interruption to compressions.

■ **If the child vomits** during CPR, roll her away from you onto her side, ensuring that her head is turned toward the floor to allow vomit to drain away. Clear the mouth, then immediately roll her onto her back again and recommence CPR.

■ **If the child is large,** or the rescuer is small, you can give chest compressions using both hands, as for an adult casualty (pp.66–67). Place one hand on the chest, cover it with your other hand, and interlock your fingers.

GIVING CHEST-COMPRESSION-ONLY CPR

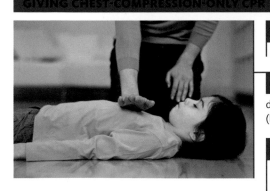

1 Kneel beside the child, level with her chest. Place the heel of one hand on the center of her chest.

2 Lean over the child with your arm straight and depress the chest by at least one third of the depth, about 2 in (5 cm), and release the pressure (but do not remove your hand).

3 Repeat compressions at a rate of at least 100 per minute until help arrives or the child shows signs of regaining consciousness, such as coughing, opening her eyes, speaking, or moving purposefully and starts to breathe normally, or you are too exhausted to continue.

PROBLEMS WITH RESCUE BREATHING

If a child's chest does not rise when you are giving rescue breaths:
■ Recheck the head tilt and chin lift
■ Recheck the mouth. Remove any obvious obstructions, but do not do a finger sweep of the mouth

Make no more than two attempts to achieve rescue breaths before repeating the chest compressions.

VARIATIONS FOR RESCUE BREATHING

There are some cases where mouth-to-mouth rescue breaths are not appropriate and you will need to use a mouth-to-nose technique.

Mouth-to-nose rescue breathing

If injuries to the mouth make it impossible to achieve a good seal, you can use the mouth-to-nose method for giving rescue breaths. With the child's mouth closed, form a tight seal with your lips around the nose and blow steadily into the casualty's nose. Then allow the mouth to fall open to let the air escape.

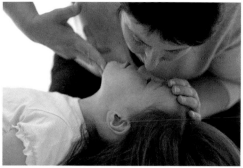

FACE SHIELDS AND POCKET MASKS

A face shield is a plastic barrier with a filter that is placed over the casualty's mouth. A pocket mask is more substantial and has a valve through which breaths are given. If you know how to use one of these aids, carry it with you and use it if you need to resuscitate a child.

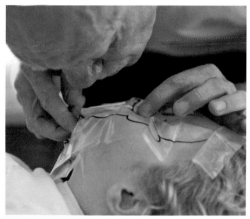

Using a face shield
Tilt the child's head back to open the airway and lift the chin. Place the plastic shield over the child's face so the filter is over her mouth. Pinch the nose, cover the child's mouth completely, and deliver breaths.

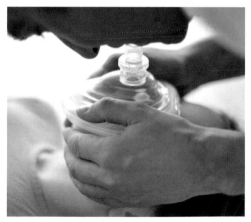

Using a pocket mask
Kneel behind the child's head. Open the airway and place the mask over the child's mouth and nose. If it is an adult-size mask, position it so that the small end is over the nose. Deliver breaths through the mouthpiece.

WHEN THE AMBULANCE ARRIVES

Tell the EMS personnel that you are a first aider and give a full report of what has happened. However, do not stop CPR while you are doing this unless they tell you to do so. Listen carefully to what they ask you to do and follow their instructions (p.23). If you have access to an AED (pp.84–87) and are trained to use it, you may have already attached it to the casualty's chest. If not, the EMS personnel will have one and attach it. You may be asked to continue with chest compressions while they do this. You will be asked to stand clear while it analyzes the casualty's heart rhythm (p.84). Do not approach the casualty again until asked to do so.

UNCONSCIOUS INFANT UNDER ONE YEAR

The following pages describe techniques that may be used for the resuscitation of an unconscious infant under one year. For a child over the age of one year, use the child resuscitation procedure (pp.72–79).

Always treat the infant from the side, the correct position for doing all the stages of resuscitation: giving chest compressions, opening the airway, and giving rescue breaths (which are together known as cardiopulmonary resuscitation, or CPR). First check responsiveness and assess for breathing; if absent, give compressions immediately. If normal breathing resumes at any stage, hold the infant in the recovery position (opposite). **Call 911 for emergency help** if any infant who becomes unconscious.

HOW TO CHECK RESPONSE

Gently tap or flick the sole of the infant's foot and call his name to see if he responds. Never shake an infant.

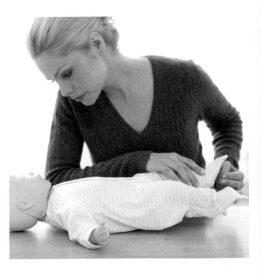

IF THERE IS NO RESPONSE
Shout for help, then start chest compressions (pp.82–83).

IF THERE IS A RESPONSE
Check and treat for life-threatening injuries. Take the infant with you to summon help if needed. Monitor and record vital signs—level of response, breathing, and pulse (pp.52–53)—until help arrives.

HOW TO OPEN THE AIRWAY

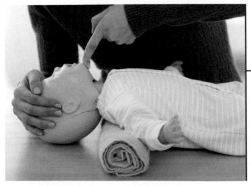

1 Place a rolled-up towel under the infant's shoulders. Place one hand on the infant's forehead and very gently tilt the head back.

2 Place one fingertip of your other hand on the point of the chin. Gently lift the point of the chin. Do not push on the soft tissues under the chin because this may block the airway.

HOW TO ASSESS FOR BREATHING

Keep the airway open and check if the infant is breathing normally. Occasional gasps (agonal breathing, p.59) do not constitute normal breathing, and if you see this, you should treat as if the infant were not breathing at all.

IF THE INFANT IS NOT BREATHING

 Ask a helper to **call 911 for emergency help.** If you are on your own, perform CPR for two minutes before making the call yourself.

Begin CPR with 30 compressions (pp.82–83).

IF THE INFANT IS BREATHING

Check for **life-threatening** injuries, such as severe bleeding, and treat if necessary.

Hold the infant in the recovery position. Monitor and record vital signs—level of response, breathing, and pulse (pp.52–53)—regularly until help arrives.

HOW TO HOLD IN RECOVERY POSITION

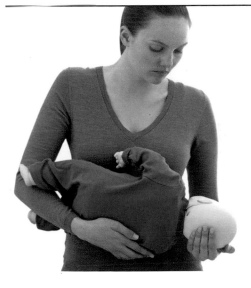

 Cradle the infant in your arms with his head tilted downward. This position prevents him from choking on his tongue or from inhaling vomit.

Monitor and record vital signs—level of response, breathing and pulse (pp.52–53) —until help arrives.

« UNCONSCIOUS INFANT UNDER ONE YEAR

HOW TO GIVE CPR

WHAT TO DO

1 Place the infant on his back on a flat surface, at waist height in front of you or on the floor, with a rolled-up towel under his shoulders.

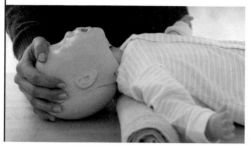

2 Place two fingertips of your lower hand on the center of the infant's chest. Press down vertically on the infant's breastbone and depress the chest by at least one-third of its depth—about 1½ in (4 cm). Release the pressure without losing the contact between your fingers and the breastbone. Repeat to give 30 compressions at a rate of at least 100 times per minute.

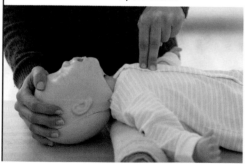

3 Open the airway by putting one hand on the infant's forehead and a fingertip of the other hand under the tip of his chin and tilting up and back as shown.

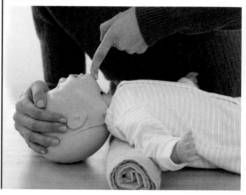

4 Pick out any visible obstructions from mouth and nose. Do not sweep the mouth with your finger looking for obstructions; this could push an object farther down.

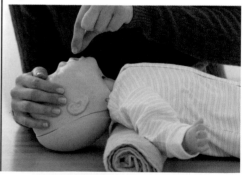

CAUTION

If you cannot achieve breaths:
- Recheck the head tilt and chin lift;
- Recheck the infant's mouth and nose and remove obvious obstructions. Do not do a finger sweep;
- Check that you have a firm seal around the mouth and nose

- Make up to two attempts to achieve rescue breaths, then continue chest compressions.
- If the infant vomits during the CPR, roll him away from you onto his side to allow the vomit to drain. Resume CPR as soon as possible

5 Take a breath. Place your lips around the infant's mouth and nose to form an airtight seal. If you cannot make a seal around the mouth and nose, close the infant's mouth and make a seal around the nose only. Blow steadily into the infant's mouth for one second; the chest should rise. Release your mouth and watch to see that the chest falls. Give a second breath.

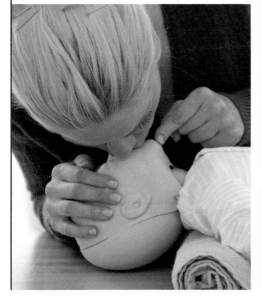

6 If you are on your own, continue alternating 30 chest compressions with TWO rescue breaths for two minutes, then stop to **call 911 for emergency help.** If help is on the way, continue CPR until emergency help arrives and takes over, the infant starts to breathe normally, or you become too exhausted to continue.

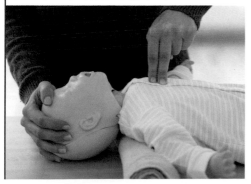

HAND POSITION

Place your fingers on the breastbone as indicated here. Make sure that you do not apply pressure over the ribs, the lower tip of the infant's breastbone or the upper abdomen.

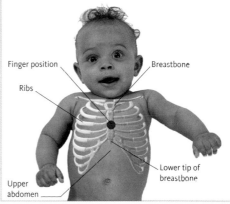

Finger position   Breastbone

Ribs

Lower tip of breastbone

Upper abdomen

CHEST-COMPRESSION-ONLY CPR

While it is better to give a combination of rescue breaths and chest compressions, if you have not had formal training in CPR, or if you are unwilling or unable to give rescue breaths, you can give chest compressions only. The dispatcher will give you instructions for chest-compression-only CPR.

CAUTION

With more than one rescuer, change every 2 minutes with minimal interruption to compressions.

HOW TO USE AN AED

CAUTION

- Make sure that no one is touching the casualty because this will interfere with the AED readings and there is a risk of electric shock.

- Do not turn off the AED or remove the pads at any point, even if the casualty appears to have recovered.

- It does not matter if the AED pads are reversed. If you put them on the wrong way, do not remove and replace them; it wastes time and the pads may not stick to the chest properly when they are reattached.

When the heart stops, a cardiac arrest has occurred. The most common cause is an abnormal rhythm of the heart, known as ventricular fibrillation. This abnormal rhythm can occur when the heart muscle is damaged as a result of a heart attack or when insufficient oxygen reaches the heart. A machine called an automated external defibrillator (AED) can be used to correct the heart rhythm by giving an electric shock. Ideally, pediatric pads should be used for children up to the age of 8, but adult pads can be used if the pediatric ones are not available. AEDs are available in many public places, including shopping centers, railroad stations, and airports. The machine analyzes the casualty's heart rhythm and shows or tells you what action to take at each stage. In most cases when an AED is called for, you will have started CPR. When the AED is brought, continue with CPR while the machine is prepared and the pads are attached to the casualty.

WHAT TO DO

1 **Switch on the AED** and take the pads out of the sealed pack. Remove or cut through clothing and wipe away sweat from the chest.

2 **Remove the backing paper** and attach the pads to the casualty's chest in the positions indicated. Place the first pad on the casualty's upper right side, just below his collarbone.

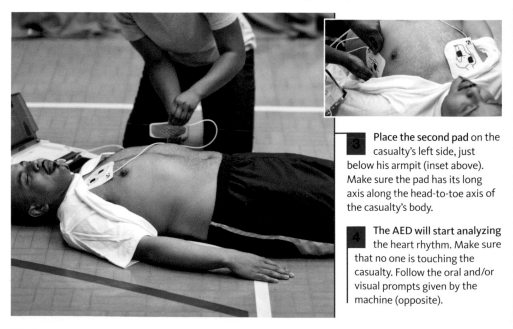

3 **Place the second pad** on the casualty's left side, just below his armpit (inset above). Make sure the pad has its long axis along the head-to-toe axis of the casualty's body.

4 **The AED will start analyzing** the heart rhythm. Make sure that no one is touching the casualty. Follow the oral and/or visual prompts given by the machine (opposite).

SEQUENCE OF AED INSTRUCTIONS

The AED will start to give you a series of visual and verbal prompts as soon as it is switched on. There are several different AED models available, each of which has voice prompts. You should always follow the prompts given by the AED that you are using until advanced emergency care is available.

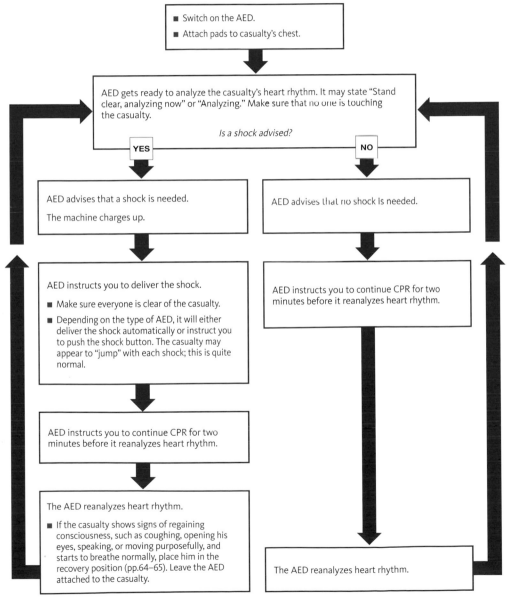

- Switch on the AED.
- Attach pads to casualty's chest.

AED gets ready to analyze the casualty's heart rhythm. It may state "Stand clear, analyzing now" or "Analyzing." Make sure that no one is touching the casualty.

Is a shock advised?

YES

NO

AED advises that a shock is needed.

The machine charges up.

AED advises that no shock is needed.

AED instructs you to deliver the shock.

- Make sure everyone is clear of the casualty.
- Depending on the type of AED, it will either deliver the shock automatically or instruct you to push the shock button. The casualty may appear to "jump" with each shock; this is quite normal.

AED instructs you to continue CPR for two minutes before it reanalyzes heart rhythm.

AED instructs you to continue CPR for two minutes before it reanalyzes heart rhythm.

The AED reanalyzes heart rhythm.

- If the casualty shows signs of regaining consciousness, such as coughing, opening his eyes, speaking, or moving purposefully, and starts to breathe normally, place him in the recovery position (pp.64–65). Leave the AED attached to the casualty.

The AED reanalyzes heart rhythm.

« HOW TO USE AN AED

CONSIDERATIONS WHEN USING AN AED

The use of an AED is occasionally complicated by underlying medical conditions, external factors, clothing, or the cause of the cardiac arrest. The safety of all concerned should always be your first consideration.

CLOTHING AND JEWELRY

Any clothing or jewelry that could interfere with pads should be removed or cut away. Normal amounts of chest hair are not a problem, but if it prevents good contact between the skin and the pads, it should be shaved off. Ensure that any metal is removed from the area where the pads will be attached. Remove clothing containing metal, such as an underwire bra.

EXTERNAL FACTORS

Water or excessive sweat on the chest can reduce the effectiveness of the shock so the chest should be dry. If a casualty is rescued from water (p.36), dry the chest before applying the AED pads.

If the casualty is unconscious following an electric shock, start CPR immediately after the contact with electricity is broken.

MEDICAL CONDITIONS

Some casualties with heart conditions have a pacemaker or an implantable cardioverter defibrillator (ICD). This should not stop you from using an AED. However, if you can see or feel a device under the chest skin, do not place the pad directly over it. If a casualty has a patch such as a nitroglycerin patch on the chest, remove it before you apply the AED.

PREGNANT CASUALTIES

There are no contraindications to using an AED during pregnancy; however, the increased breast size may present some problems. Therefore, to place the AED pads correctly, you may need to move one or both breasts. This must be carried out with respect and dignity.

POSITIONING AED PADS ON CHILDREN

Standard adult AEDs can be used on children over the age of eight years. For children between the ages of one and eight, the smaller-sized, pediatric pads are preferred if they are available. If not, a standard AED and adult pads can be used.

> **CAUTION**
>
> A manual defibrillator is preferred for infants younger than one year of age, but if none is available, use an AED with pediatric pads.

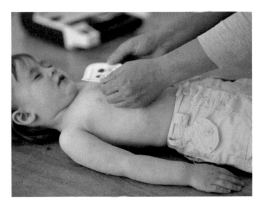

Positioning pediatric AED pads
Place one pad in the center of the child's back. Then place the second pad over the center of the child's chest. Make sure both pads are vertical. Connect the pads to the AED and proceed as described on p.85.

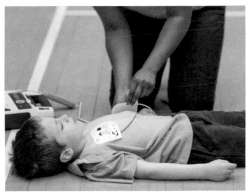

Using AED pads on a larger child
Place the pads on the child's chest as for an adult—one on the child's upper right side, just below his collarbone, and the second pad on the child's left side, just below the armpit. Make sure the long axis of the pad is along the head-to-toe axis of the child's body.

HANDING OVER TO THE EMERGENCY SERVICES

When the emergency services arrive continue to resuscitate the child until they take over from you. They need to know:
- **Casualty's present status;** for example, unconscious and not breathing
- **Number of shocks** you have delivered
- **When the casualty collapsed** and the length of time he has been unconscious
- **Any relevant history,** if known

If the casualty recovers at any point, leave the AED pads attached to his chest. Ensure that any used materials from the AED cabinet are disposed of as clinical waste (p.238). Inform the relevant person what has been taken out of the cabinet because it will need to be replaced.

87

5

Oxygen is essential to life. Every time we inhale, air containing oxygen enters the lungs. This oxygen is then transferred to the blood, to be transported around the body. Breathing and the exchange of oxygen and carbon dioxide (a waste product from body tissues) are described as "respiration." The structures within the body that enable us to breathe—the air passages and the lungs—together make up the respiratory system, and work with the heart and circulatory system.

Respiration can be impaired in several different ways. The airways may be blocked, causing choking or suffocation; the exchange of oxygen and carbon dioxide in the lungs may be affected by the inhalation of smoke or fumes; lung function may be impaired by chest injury; or the breathing mechanism may be affected by conditions such as asthma. Anxiety can also cause breathing difficulties. Problems with respiration can be life-threatening and need urgent first aid.

AIMS AND OBJECTIVES

- To assess the casualty's condition.
- To identify and remove the cause of the problem and provide fresh air.
- To comfort and reassure the casualty.
- To maintain an open airway, check breathing and be prepared to resuscitate if necessary.
- To obtain medical help if necessary. **Call 911 for emergency help** if you suspect a serious illness or injury.

RESPIRATORY
PROBLEMS

THE RESPIRATORY SYSTEM

This system comprises the mouth, nose, windpipe (trachea), lungs, and pulmonary blood vessels. Respiration involves the process of breathing and the exchange of gases (oxygen and carbon dioxide) in the lungs and in cells throughout the body.

We inhale air to take oxygen into the lungs, and we exhale to expel the waste gas, carbon dioxide, which is a by-product of respiration. When we inhale, air is drawn through the nose and mouth into the airway and the lungs. In the lungs, oxygen is taken from air sacs (alveoli) into the pulmonary capillaries. At the same time, carbon dioxide is released from the capillaries into the alveoli. Carbon dioxide is then expelled as we exhale. An average man's lungs can hold more than 10 pints (6 liters) of air; a woman's lungs can hold less than 9 pints (5 liters) of air.

Structure of the respiratory system
The lungs form the central part of the respiratory system. Together with the circulatory system, they perform the vital function of gas exchange in order to distribute oxygen around the body and remove carbon dioxide.

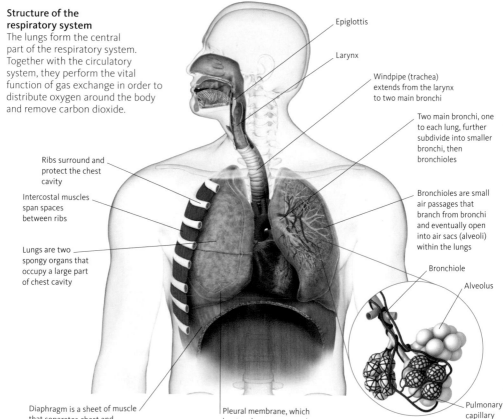

Epiglottis

Larynx

Windpipe (trachea) extends from the larynx to two main bronchi

Two main bronchi, one to each lung, further subdivide into smaller bronchi, then bronchioles

Bronchioles are small air passages that branch from bronchi and eventually open into air sacs (alveoli) within the lungs

Ribs surround and protect the chest cavity

Intercostal muscles span spaces between ribs

Lungs are two spongy organs that occupy a large part of chest cavity

Bronchiole

Alveolus

Diaphragm is a sheet of muscle that separates chest and abdominal cavities

Pleural membrane, which has two layers separated by a lubricating fluid, surrounds and protects each of the lungs

Pulmonary capillary

Gas exchange in air sacs
A network of tiny blood vessels (capillaries) surrounds each air sac (alveolus). The thin walls of both structures allow oxygen to diffuse into the blood and carbon dioxide to leave it.

HOW BREATHING WORKS

The breathing process consists of the actions of breathing in (inspiration) and breathing out (expiration), followed by a pause. Pressure differences between the lungs and the air outside the body determine whether air is drawn in or expelled. When the air pressure in the lungs is lower than outside, air is drawn in; when pressure is higher, air is expelled. The pressure within the lungs is altered by the movements of the two main sets of muscles involved in breathing: the intercostal muscles and the diaphragm.

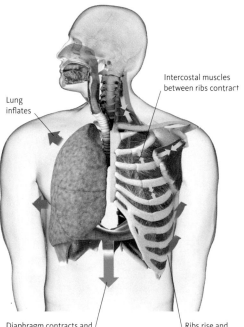

Lung inflates

Intercostal muscles between ribs contract

Diaphragm contracts and moves down

Ribs rise and swing outward

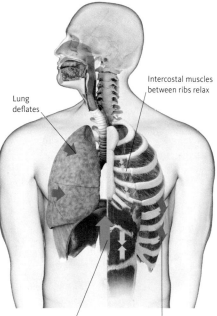

Lung deflates

Intercostal muscles between ribs relax

Diaphragm returns to domed position

Ribs move down and inward

Inhaling
The intercostal muscles (the muscles between the ribs) and the diaphragm contract, causing the ribs to move up and out, the chest cavity to expand, and the lungs to expand to fill the space. As a result, the pressure inside the lungs is reduced, and air is drawn into the lungs.

Exhaling
The intercostal muscles relax, and the rib cage returns to its resting position, while the diaphragm relaxes and resumes its domed shape. As a result, the chest cavity becomes smaller, and pressure inside the lungs increases. Air flows out of the lungs to be exhaled.

HOW BREATHING IS CONTROLLED

Breathing is regulated by a group of nerve cells in the brain called the respiratory center. This center responds to changes in the level of carbon dioxide in the blood. When the level rises, the respiratory center reacts by stimulating the intercostal muscles and the diaphragm to contract, and a breath occurs. Our breathing rate can be altered consciously under normal conditions or in response to abnormal levels of carbon dioxide, low levels of oxygen, or with stress, exercise, injury, or illness.

HYPOXIA

RECOGNITION

In moderate and severe hypoxia, there may be:

- Rapid breathing
- Breathing that is distressed or gasping
- Difficulty speaking
- Gray-blue skin (cyanosis). At first, this is more obvious in the extremities, such as lips, nailbeds, and earlobes, but as the hypoxia worsens cyanosis affects the rest of the body
- Anxiety
- Restlessness
- Headache
- Cessation of breathing if the hypoxia is not quickly reversed

This condition arises when there is insufficient oxygen in the body tissues. There are a number of causes of hypoxia, ranging from suffocation, choking, or poisoning to impaired lung or brain function. The condition is accompanied by a variety of symptoms, depending on the degree of hypoxia. If not treated quickly, hypoxia is potentially fatal because a sufficient level of oxygen is vital for the normal function of all the body organs and tissues, but especially the brain.

In a healthy person, the amount of oxygen in the air is more than adequate for the body tissues to function normally. However, in an injured or ill person, a reduction in oxygen reaching the tissues results in deterioration of body function.

Mild hypoxia reduces a casualty's ability to think clearly, but the body responds to this by increasing the rate and depth of breathing (p.91). However, if the oxygen supply to the brain cells is cut off for as little as three to four minutes, the brain cells will begin to die. All the conditions covered in this chapter can result in hypoxia.

INJURIES OR CONDITIONS CAUSING LOW BLOOD OXYGEN (HYPOXIA)	
INJURY OR CONDITION	**CAUSES**
Insufficient oxygen in inspired air	■ Suffocation by smoke or gas ■ Changes in atmospheric pressure, for example, at high altitude or in a depressurized aircraft
Airway obstruction	■ Blocking or swelling of the airway ■ Hanging or strangulation ■ Something covering the mouth and nose ■ Asthma ■ Choking ■ Anaphylaxis
Conditions affecting the chest wall	■ Crushing, for example, by falling earth or sand or pressure from a crowd ■ Chest wall injury with multiple rib fractures or constricting burns
Impaired lung function	■ Lung injury ■ Collapsed lung ■ Lung infections, such as pneumonia
Damage to the brain or nerves that control respiration	■ A head injury or stroke that damages the breathing center in the brain ■ Some forms of poisoning ■ Paralysis of nerves controlling the muscles of breathing, as in spinal cord injury
Impaired oxygen uptake by the tissues	■ Carbon monoxide or cyanide poisoning ■ Shock

SEE ALSO Anaphylactic shock p.223 | Asthma p.102 | Burns to the airway p.177 | Croup p.103 | Drowning p.100 | Hanging and strangulation p.97 | Inhalation of fumes pp.98–99 | Penetrating chest wound pp.104–05 | Stroke pp.212–13

AIRWAY OBSTRUCTION

The airway may be obstructed externally or internally, for example, by an object that is stuck at the back of the throat (pp.94–96). The main causes of obstruction are:

- **Inhalation** of an object, such as food
- **Blockage** by the tongue, blood, or vomit while a casualty is unconscious (p.59)
- **Internal swelling** of the throat occurring with burns, scalds, stings, or anaphylaxis
- **Injuries** to the face or jaw
- **An asthma attack** in which the small airways in the lungs constrict (p.102)
- **External pressure** on the neck, as in hanging or strangulation
- **Peanuts,** which can swell up when in contact with body fluids. These pose a particular danger in young children because they can completely block the airway

Try to encourage a toddler to cough up the object; an older child can be treated with abdominal thrusts as shown on p.95. Airway obstruction requires prompt action; be prepared to give chest compressions and rescue breaths if the child loses consciousness (Unconscious child, pp.76–79).

CAUTION

- If the casualty is unconscious, look for normal breathing and, if not, begin CPR with compressions (pp.54–87).

RECOGNITION

- Features of hypoxia (opposite)
- Difficulty speaking and breathing
- Noisy breathing in partial airway obstruction
- Silence or minimal, high-pitched sounds if complete or near complete obstruction
- Red, puffy face
- Signs of distress from the casualty, who may point to the throat or grasp the neck

YOUR AIMS

- To remove the obstruction
- To restore normal breathing
- To arrange removal to the hospital

SEE ALSO Asthma **p.102** | Burns to the airway **p.177** | Choking adult **p.94** | Choking child **p.95** | Choking infant **p.96** | Drowning **p.100** | Hanging and strangulation **p.97** | Inhalation of fumes **pp.98–99**

CHOKING ADULT

RECOGNITION

Ask the casualty:
"Are you choking?"

Mild obstruction:
- Casualty able to speak, cough, and breathe

Severe obstruction:
- Casualty unable to speak, cough or breathe, with eventual loss of consciousness

YOUR AIMS

- To remove the obstruction
- To arrange urgent removal to the hospital if necessary

A foreign object that is stuck in the throat may block it and cause laryngeal spasm. If blockage of the airway is mild, the casualty should be able to clear it; if it is severe, she will be unable to speak, cough, or breathe, and will eventually lose consciousness. If she loses consciousness, the throat muscles may relax and the airway may open enough to do rescue breathing. Be prepared to begin chest compressions and rescue breaths.

WHAT TO DO

1 If the casualty is breathing, encourage her to continue coughing. If she is not coughing and not able to breathe, she is choking. Go to step 2.

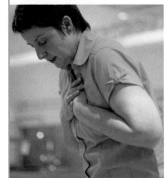

2 Stand behind the casualty with one leg back and the other between the casualty's legs, and put both arms around the upper part of her abdomen. Clench your fist with your thumb on top of your index finger and place it between the navel and the bottom of her breastbone. Grasp your fist firmly with your other hand. Thrust sharply inward and upward until the object is dislodged or the casualty becomes unconscious.

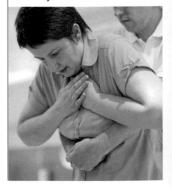

3 If the casualty loses consciousness, carefully support her to the floor, immediately **call 911 for emergency help** or send someone to do so, then begin CPR with chest compressions (pp.66–67). Each time the airway is opened during CPR, look for an object in the casualty's mouth and, if seen, remove it.

4 **If the obstruction** still has not cleared, continue CPR until help arrives.

CHOKING CHILD ONE YEAR TO PUBERTY

Young children especially are prone to choking. A child may choke on food, or may put small objects into her mouth and cause a blockage of the airway.

    If a child is choking, you need to act quickly. If she loses consciousness, the throat muscles may relax and the airway may open enough to do rescue breathing. Be prepared to begin rescue breaths and chest compressions.

WHAT TO DO

1 If the child is breathing, encourage her to continue coughing. If she is not coughing and not able to breathe, she is choking. Go to step 2.

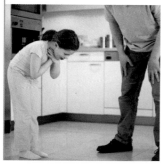

2 **Put your arms** around the child's upper abdomen. Place your fist between the navel and the bottom of her breastbone, and grasp it with your other hand. Pull sharply inward and upward until the object is dislodged or the child becomes unconscious.

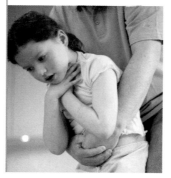

RECOGNITION

Ask the child: "Are you choking?"

Mild obstruction:
- Child able to speak, cough, and breathe

Severe obstruction:
- Child unable to speak, cough or breathe, with eventual loss of consciousness.

YOUR AIMS

- To remove the obstruction
- To arrange urgent removal to the hospital if necessary

3 If the child becomes unresponsive, carefully support her to the ground and start CPR with chest compressions (pp.76–77). After 30 compressions, open the airway and look in her mouth. If a foreign body is seen, remove it but do not perform blind finger sweeps. Then attempt to give two breaths and continue with cycles of chest compressions and ventilations until the object is expelled.

4 After two minutes, if no one has already done so, the obstruction still has not cleared or the child has not regained consciousness, **call 911 for emergency help**. Then continue CPR until help arrives.

CHOKING INFANT UNDER ONE YEAR

CAUTION

- If the infant loses consciousness at any stage, assess breathing (pp.80–81). If the infant is not breathing, begin CPR with chest compressions (pp.82–83), then open the airway and remove any obvious foreign objects, give two rescue breaths if possible, and repeat compressions.

- Seek medical advice for any infant who has been given chest compressions.

RECOGNITION

Mild obstruction:
- Infant able to cough, but has difficulty crying or making any other noise

Severe obstruction:
- Unable to make any noise, or breathe, with eventual loss of consciousness

YOUR AIMS

- To remove the obstruction
- To arrange urgent removal to the hospital if necessary

An infant is more likely to choke on food or small objects than an adult. The infant will rapidly become distressed, and you need to act quickly to clear any obstruction. If the infant loses consciousness, the throat muscles may relax and the airway may open enough to do rescue breathing. Be prepared to begin chest compressions and rescue breaths.

WHAT TO DO

1 If the infant is distressed, is unable to cry, cough, or breathe, lay him face down along your forearm, with his head low, and support his back and head. Give up to five back blows, with the heel of your hand.

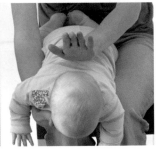

2 If back blows fail to clear the obstruction, turn the infant onto his back and give chest compressions. Using two fingers, push against the infant's breastbone, in the nipple line.

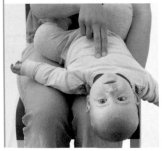

3 Perform up to five chest compressions. The aim is to relieve the obstruction with each chest compression rather than necessarily doing all five.

4 Check the infant's mouth; remove any obvious obstructions with your fingertips. Do not sweep the mouth with your finger because this may push the object farther down the throat. Repeat steps 1–4 until the object clears or the infant loses consciousness.

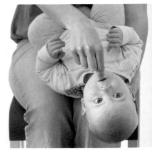

5 If the obstruction has not cleared and he becomes unconscious, **call 911 for emergency help,** then start CPR with chest compressions (pp.82–83). Continue until help arrives.

HANGING AND STRANGULATION

If pressure is exerted on the outside of the neck, the airway is squeezed and the flow of air to the lungs is cut off. The main causes of such pressure are:

- **Hanging**—suspension of the body by a noose around the neck;
- **Strangulation**—constriction or squeezing around the neck or throat.

Sometimes, hanging or strangulation may occur accidentally—for example, by ties or clothing becoming caught in machinery. Hanging may cause a broken neck; for this reason, a casualty in this situation must be handled extremely carefully.

WHAT TO DO

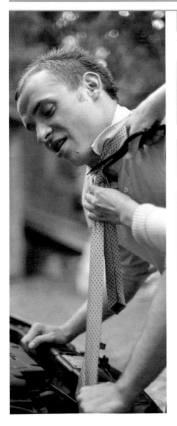

1 Quickly remove any constriction from around the casualty's neck.

2 If the casualty is hanging, support the body while you relieve the constriction. Be aware that the body will be very heavy if he is unconscious.

3 If conscious, help the casualty to lie down while you support his head and neck.

4 Call 911 for emergency help, even if he appears to recover fully. Monitor and record his vital signs—level of response, breathing, and pulse (pp.52–53)—until help arrives.

RECOGNITION

- A constricting article around the neck
- Marks around the casualty's neck
- Rapid, difficult breathing; impaired consciousness; gray–blue skin (cyanosis)
- Congestion of the face, with prominent veins: may have tiny red spots on the face or eyelids, or red areas in the whites of the eyes

YOUR AIMS

- To restore adequate breathing
- To arrange urgent removal to the hospital

INHALATION OF FUMES

The inhalation of smoke, gases (such as carbon monoxide), or toxic vapors can be lethal. A casualty who has inhaled fumes is likely to have low levels of oxygen in his body tissues (hypoxia, p.92) and therefore needs urgent medical attention. Do not attempt to carry out a rescue if it is likely to put your own life at risk; fumes that have built up in a confined space will quickly overcome anyone who is not wearing protective equipment.

SMOKE INHALATION

Any person who has been enclosed in a confined space during a fire should be assumed to have inhaled smoke. Smoke from burning plastics, foam padding, and synthetic wall coverings is likely to contain poisonous fumes. Casualties who have suffered from fume inhalation should also be examined for other injuries caused by the fire, such as external burns.

INHALATION OF CARBON MONOXIDE

Carbon monoxide is a poisonous gas that is hard to detect because it has no taste or smell. The gas acts directly on red blood cells, preventing them from carrying oxygen to the body tissues. If carbon monoxide is inhaled in large quantities—for example, from smoke or vehicle exhaust fumes in a confined space—it can very quickly prove fatal. Lengthy exposure to even a small amount of carbon monoxide—for example, due to a leakage of fumes from a defective heater or flue—may also prove fatal.

EFFECTS OF FUME INHALATION		
FUMES	**SOURCE**	**EFFECTS**
Carbon monoxide	■ Exhaust fumes of motor vehicles ■ Smoke from most fires ■ Back-drafts from blocked chimney flues ■ Emissions from defective gas or kerosene heaters and poorly maintained heaters ■ Disposable or portable barbeques used in a confined space	Prolonged exposure to low levels: ■ Headache ■ Confusion ■ Aggression ■ Nausea and vomiting ■ Incontinence Brief exposure to high levels: ■ Gray-blue skin coloration ■ Rapid, difficult breathing ■ Impaired consciousness, leading to unconsciousness
Smoke	■ Fires: smoke is a bigger killer than fire itself. Smoke is low in oxygen (which is used up by the burning of the fire) and may contain toxic fumes from burning materials	■ Rapid, noisy, and difficult breathing ■ Coughing and wheezing ■ Burning in the nose or mouth ■ Soot around the mouth and nose ■ Unconsciousness
Carbon dioxide	■ Tends to accumulate and become dangerously concentrated in deep enclosed spaces, such as coal pits, wells, and underground tanks	■ Breathlessness ■ Headache ■ Confusion ■ Unconsciousness
Solvents and fuels	■ Glues ■ Cleaning fluids ■ Lighter fuels ■ Camping gas and propane-fueled stoves (Solvent abusers may use a plastic bag to concentrate the vapor, especially with glues)	■ Headache and vomiting ■ Impaired consciousness ■ Airway obstruction from using a plastic bag or from choking on vomit may result in death ■ Solvent abuse is a potential cause of cardiac arrest

WHAT TO DO

1 **Call 911 for emergency help.** Tell the dispatcher that you suspect fume inhalation.

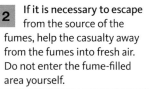

3 **Support the casualty** and encourage him to breathe normally. If the casualty's clothing is still burning, try to extinguish the flames (p.33). Treat any obvious burns (pp.174–77) or other injuries.

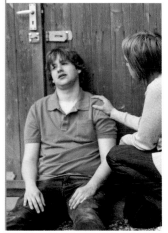

2 **If it is necessary to escape** from the source of the fumes, help the casualty away from the fumes into fresh air. Do not enter the fume-filled area yourself.

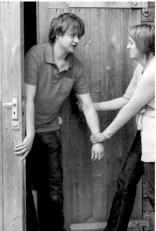

4 **Stay with the casualty** until help arrives. Monitor and record the casualty's vital signs—level of response, breathing, and pulse (pp.52–53)—until help arrives.

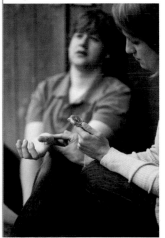

CAUTION

- If the casualty is in a garage filled with vehicle exhaust fumes, open the doors wide and let the gas escape before you enter.
- If the casualty is found unconscious and is not breathing normally, begin CPR with chest compressions (pp.54–87).

YOUR AIMS

- To restore adequate breathing
- To **call 911 for emergency help** and obtain urgent medical attention

SEE ALSO Burns to the airway **p.177** | Fires **pp.32–33** | Hypoxia **p.92** | The unconscious casualty **pp.54–87**

DROWNING

Drowning can result in death from hypothermia due to immersion in cold water, sudden cardiac arrest due to cold water, spasm of the throat blocking the airway and/or inhalation of water and consequent airway obstruction.

A casualty rescued from a drowning incident should always receive medical attention even if he seems to have recovered at the time. Any water entering the lungs causes them to become irritated, and the air passages may begin to swell several hours later—a condition known as secondary drowning. The casualty may also need to be treated for hypothermia (pp.186–88).

YOUR AIMS

- To restore adequate breathing
- To keep the casualty warm
- To arrange urgent removal to the hospital

WHAT TO DO

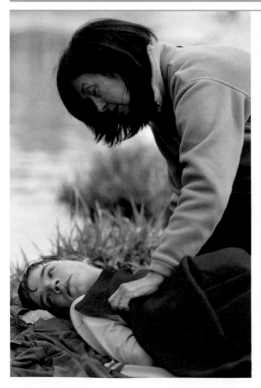

1 If you have rescued the casualty from the water, help him lie down on a rug or coat with his head lower than the rest of the body so that water can drain from his mouth. This reduces the risk of inhaling water (p.36).

2 Treat the casualty for hypothermia; replace wet clothing with dry clothes if possible and cover him with dry blankets or coats. If the casualty is fully conscious, give him a warm drink.

3 **Call 911 for emergency help** even if he appears to recover fully because of the risk of secondary drowning. Monitor and record his vital signs—level of response, breathing, and pulse (pp.52–53)—until help arrives.

4 If the casualty is unconscious and you are on your own, give CPR for two minutes before you **call 911 for emergency help.**

5 If an unconscious casualty starts to breathe, treat him for hypothermia by covering him with warm clothes and blankets. If he recovers, replace his wet clothes with dry ones if possible and cover him with warm clothes and blankets. Monitor and record vital signs—breathing, pulse and level of response (pp.52–53)—until help arrives.

HYPERVENTILATION

This is commonly a manifestation of acute anxiety and may accompany a panic attack. It may occur in individuals who have recently experienced an emotional upset or those with a history of panic attacks.

The unnaturally fast or deep breathing of hyperventilation causes an increased loss of carbon dioxide from the blood, which leads to chemical changes within the blood. These changes result in symptoms such as dizziness, and trembling, as well as tingling in the hands. As breathing returns to normal, these symptoms will gradually subside.

WHAT TO DO

1 When speaking to the casualty, be firm, but kind and reassuring. If possible, lead the casualty away to a quiet place where she may be able to regain control of her breathing more easily and quickly. If this is not possible, ask any bystanders to leave.

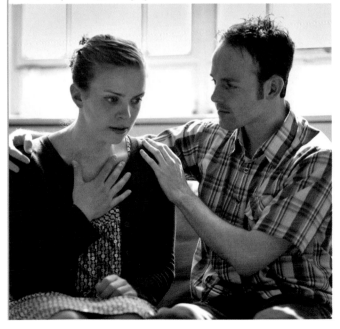

2 Encourage the casualty to seek medical advice on preventing and controlling panic attacks in the future.

RECOGNITION

- Unnaturally fast breathing
- Fast pulse rate
- Apprehension

There may also be:

- Attention-seeking behavior
- Dizziness or faintness
- Trembling, sweating, and dry mouth, or marked tingling in the hands
- Tingling and cramps in the hands and feet and around the mouth

YOUR AIMS

- To remove the casualty from the cause of distress
- To reassure the casualty and calm her down

ASTHMA

RECOGNITION

- Difficulty breathing
- Wheezing
- Difficulty speaking, leading to short sentences and whispering
- Coughing
- Distress and anxiety
- Features of hypoxia (p.92), such as a gray-blue tinge to the lips, earlobes, and nailbeds (cyanosis)
- Exhaustion in a severe attack. If the attack worsens, the casualty may stop breathing and lose consciousness

YOUR AIMS

- To ease breathing
- To obtain medical help if necessary

In an asthma attack, the muscles of the air passages in the lungs go into spasm. As a result, the airways become narrowed, which makes breathing difficult.

Sometimes, there is a recognized trigger for an attack, such as an allergy, a cold, a particular drug, or cigarette smoke. At other times, there is no obvious trigger. Many sufferers have sudden attacks.

People with asthma may be treated, depending on the severity of their condition, with rescue inhalers or nebulizers on a regular basis. They can usually deal with their own attacks by using their inhaler at the first sign of an attack, but may need help and encouragement.

WHAT TO DO

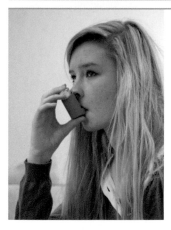

1 Keep calm and reassure the casualty. Get her to take her usual dose of her inhaler; use a spacer if she has one. Ask her to breathe slowly and deeply.

2 Sit her down in the position she finds most comfortable; do not let her lie down.

3 A mild attack should ease in a few minutes. If it does not, ask the casualty to take another dose from her inhaler.

4 Call 911 for emergency help if the attack is severe and any of the following occur: the inhaler has no effect; the casualty is getting worse; breathlessness makes talking hard; she becomes exhausted.

5 Help the casualty use her inhaler as required. Monitor her vital signs—level of response, breathing, and pulse (pp.52–53)—until help arrives.

SPECIAL CASE USING A SPACER

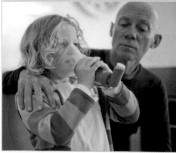

A spacer device can be fitted to an asthma inhaler to help a casualty inhale the medication more effectively. They are especially useful when giving medication to young children.

CROUP

Croup can cause an attack of breathing difficulty in young children. It is caused by a viral infection in the windpipe and larynx. Although croup can be alarming, it usually passes without lasting harm. Attacks of croup usually occur at night and are made worse if the child is crying and distressed.

If an attack of croup persists, or is severe, and accompanied by fever, call for emergency help. There is a small risk that the child is suffering from a rare, crouplike condition called epiglottitis, in which the epiglottis (p.90), a small, flaplike structure in the throat, becomes infected and swollen and may block the airway completely. Most children are now immunized against the bacterium that causes epiglottitis.

CAUTION

- Do not put your fingers down the child's throat. This can cause the throat muscles to go into spasm and block the airway.

RECOGNITION

- Distressed breathing in a young child.

There may also be:

- A short, barking cough
- A rasping noise, especially on inhaling (stridor)
- Croaky voice
- Blue-gray skin (cyanosis)
- In severe cases, the child uses muscles around the nose, neck, and upper arms in trying to breathe

Suspect epiglottitis if:

- A child is in respiratory distress and not improving
- The child has a high temperature

YOUR AIMS

- To comfort and support the child
- To obtain medical help if necessary

WHAT TO DO

1 Sit your child on your knee, supporting her back. Calmly reassure the child. Try not to panic because this will only alarm her, which is likely to make the attack worse.

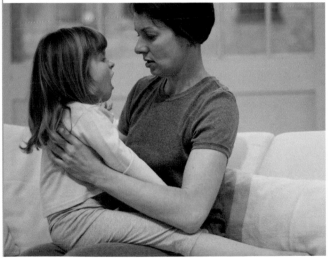

2 If it is safe to do so, create a steamy atmosphere. Take the child into the bathroom and run a hot faucet or shower, or boil some water in the kitchen. Keep the child away from hot running water or steam.

3 Call medical help or, if the croup is severe, **call 911 for emergency help.** Keep monitoring her vital signs—level of response, breathing, and pulse (pp.52–53)—until help arrives.

PENETRATING CHEST WOUND

- Difficult and painful breathing, possibly rapid, shallow, and uneven
- Casualty feels acute sense of alarm
- Features of hypoxia (p.92), including gray-blue skin coloration (cyanosis)

There may also be:

- Coughed-up frothy, red blood
- A crackling feeling of the skin around the site of the wound, caused by air collecting in the tissues
- Blood bubbling out of the wound
- Sound of air being sucked into the chest as the casualty inhales
- Veins in the neck becoming prominent

YOUR AIMS

- To seal the wound and maintain breathing
- To minimize shock
- To arrange urgent removal to the hospital

The heart and lungs, and the major blood vessels around them, lie in the chest, protected by the breastbone and the rib cage. The rib cage also extends far enough down to protect organs such as the liver and spleen in the upper part of the abdomen.

If a sharp object penetrates the chest wall, there may be severe damage to the organs in the chest and the upper abdomen and this may lead to shock. The lungs are particularly susceptible to injury, either by being damaged themselves or from wounds that perforate the two-layered membrane (pleura) that surrounds and protects each lung. Air can then enter between the membranes and exert pressure on the lung, and the lung may collapse—a condition called pneumothorax.

Pressure around the affected lung may build up to such an extent that it affects the uninjured lung, and the casualty becomes increasingly breathless. In a tension pneumothorax, this pressure buildup may prevent the heart from refilling with blood properly, impairing the circulation and causing shock. Sometimes, blood collects in the pleural cavity (a hemothorax) and puts pressure on the lungs.

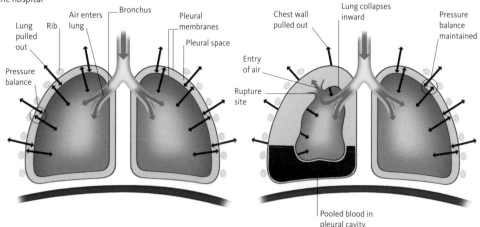

Normal breathing
The lungs inflate by being pulled out as they "suck" onto the chest wall. Pressure is maintained within the fluid-filled pleural space.

Collapsed (right) lung
Air from the right lung enters the surrounding pleural space and changes the pressure balance. The lung shrinks away from the chest wall.

WHAT TO DO

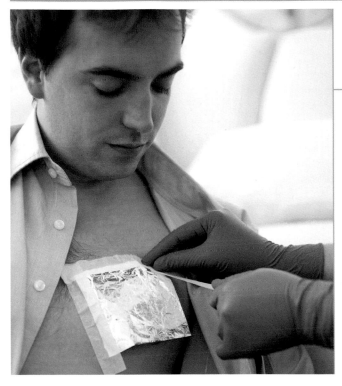

1 Help the casualty sit down. Encourage him to lean toward the injured side and cover the wound with the palm of his hand.

2 Cover the wound and surrounding area with a plastic bag or foil. Secure firmly with adhesive tape on four sides but leave one lower corner untaped.

3 Call 911 for emergency help. While waiting for help, continue to support the casualty in the same position as long as he remains conscious.

4 Monitor and record the casualty's vital signs—level of response, breathing, and pulse (pp.52–53)—until emergency help arrives.

SPECIAL CASE IF THE CASUALTY IS UNCONSCIOUS

If the casualty is unconscious, assess for normal breathing. If absent, begin CPR with chest compressions (pp.54–87). If you need to place a breathing casualty in the recovery position, roll him onto his injured side to help the healthy lung work effectively (p.64).

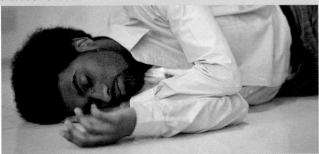

6

The heart and blood vessels are collectively known as the circulatory (cardiovascular) system. This system keeps the body supplied with blood, which carries oxygen and nutrients to all body tissues. The circulatory system may be disrupted by either severe internal or external bleeding or fluid loss, for example from burns (pp.174–79). The techniques described in this section show how you can help maintain an adequate blood supply to the heart and brain following injury or illness affecting the circulatory system.

A break in the skin or the internal body surfaces is known as a wound. Wounds can be daunting, particularly if there is a lot of bleeding, but prompt action reduces the amount of blood loss and minimizes shock. Treatments for all circulatory conditions and types of wounds are covered in this chapter.

AIMS AND OBJECTIVES

- To assess the casualty's condition quickly and calmly.
- To control blood loss by applying pressure and elevating the injured part.
- To minimize the risk of shock.
- To comfort and reassure the casualty.
- To **call 911 for emergency help** if you suspect a serious injury or illness.
- To be aware of your own needs, including the need to protect yourself against blood-borne infections.

WOUNDS AND CIRCULATION

THE HEART AND BLOOD VESSELS

The heart and the blood vessels make up the circulatory system. These structures supply the body with a constant flow of blood, which brings oxygen and nutrients to the tissues and carries waste products away.

Blood is pumped around the body by rhythmic contractions (beats) of the heart muscle. The blood runs through a network of vessels, divided into three types: arteries, veins, and capillaries. The force that is exerted by the blood flow through the main arteries is called blood pressure. The pressure varies with the strength and phase of the heartbeat, the elasticity of the arterial walls, and the volume and thickness of the blood.

How blood circulates
Oxygenated blood passes from the lungs to the heart, then travels to body tissues via the arteries. Blood that has given up its oxygen (deoxygenated blood) returns to the heart through the veins.

Carotid artery

Jugular vein

Brachial vein

Brachial artery

Aorta carries oxygenated blood to body tissues

Pulmonary arteries carry deoxygenated blood to lungs

Vena cava carries deoxygenated blood from body tissues to heart

Pulmonary veins carry oxygenated blood from lungs to heart

Heart pumps blood around body

Radial artery

Femoral artery

Radial vein

Small artery (arteriole)

Femoral vein

Capillary

Small vein (venule)

Aorta

Pulmonary artery

Superior vena cava

Coronary artery

Heart muscle

Capillary networks
A network of fine blood vessels (capillaries) links arteries and veins within body tissues. Oxygen and nutrients pass from the blood into the tissues; waste products pass from the tissues into the blood, through capillaries.

Inferior vena cava

KEY
■ Vessels carrying oxygenated blood
■ Vessels carrying deoxygenated blood

The heart
This muscular organ pumps blood around the body and then to the lungs to pick up oxygen. Coronary blood vessels supply the heart muscle with oxygen and nutrients.

HOW THE HEART FUNCTIONS

The heart pumps blood by muscular contractions called heartbeats, which are controlled by electrical impulses generated in the heart. Each beat has three phases: diastole, when the blood enters the heart; atrial systole, when it is squeezed out of the atria (collecting chambers); and ventricular systole, when blood leaves the heart.

In diastole, the heart relaxes. Oxygenated blood from the lungs flows through the pulmonary veins into the left atrium. Blood that has given up its oxygen to body tissues (deoxygenated blood) flows from the venae cavae (large veins that enter the heart) into the right atrium.

In atrial systole, the two atria contract and the valves between the atria and the ventricles (pumping chambers) open so that blood flows into the ventricles.

During ventricular systole, the ventricles contract. The thick-walled left ventricle forces blood into the aorta (main artery), which carries it to the rest of the body. The right ventricle pumps blood into the pulmonary arteries, which carry it to the lungs to collect more oxygen.

Ascending aorta carries blood to upper body

Superior vena cava carries blood from upper body

Pulmonary arteries carry deoxygenated blood to lungs

Left atrium

Right atrium

Valve

Right ventricle

Left ventricle

Inferior vena cava carries blood from lower body

Descending aorta carries blood to lower body

Blood flow through the heart
The heart's right side pumps deoxygenated blood from the body to the lungs. The left side pumps oxygenated blood to the body via the aorta.

KEY
- ■ Vessels carrying oxygenated blood
- ■ Vessels carrying deoxygenated blood

COMPOSITION OF BLOOD

There are about 10 pints (5 liters), or 1 pint per 14 pounds of body weight (1 liter per 13 kg), of blood in the average adult body. Roughly 55 percent of the blood is clear yellow fluid (plasma). In this fluid are suspended the red and white blood cells and the platelets, all of which make up the remaining 45 percent.

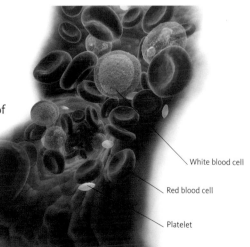

White blood cell

Red blood cell

Platelet

The blood cells
Red blood cells contain hemoglobin, a red pigment that enables the cells to carry oxygen. White blood cells play a role in defending the body against infection. Platelets help blood clot.

BLEEDING AND TYPES OF WOUND

When a blood vessel is damaged, the vessel constricts, and a series of chemical reactions occur to form a blood clot—a "plug" over the damaged area (below). If large blood vessels are torn or severed, uncontrolled blood loss may occur before clotting can take place, and shock (pp.112–13) may develop.

TYPES OF BLEEDING

Bleeding (hemorrhage) is characterized by the type of blood vessel that is damaged. Arteries carry oxygenated blood under pressure from the heart. If an artery is damaged, bleeding will be profuse. Blood will spurt out with each heartbeat. If a main artery is severed, the volume of circulating blood will fall rapidly.

Blood from veins, having given up its oxygen into the tissues, is darker red. It is under less pressure than arterial blood, but vein walls can widen greatly and the blood can "pool" inside them (varicose vein). If a large or varicose vein is damaged, blood will gush from it profusely.

Bleeding from capillaries occurs with any wound. At first, bleeding may be brisk, but blood loss is usually slight. A blow may rupture capillaries under the skin, causing bleeding into the tissues (bruising).

HOW WOUNDS HEAL

When a blood vessel is severed or damaged, it constricts (narrows) in order to prevent excessive amounts of blood from escaping. Injured tissue cells at the site of the wound, together with specialized blood cells called platelets, then trigger a series of chemical reactions that result in the formation of a substance that forms a mesh. This mesh traps blood cells to make a blood clot. The clot releases a fluid known as serum, which contains antibodies and specialized cells; this serum begins the process of repairing the damaged area.

At first, the blood clot is a jellylike mass. Fibroblast cells form a plug within the clot. Later, this dries into a crust (scab) that seals and protects the site of the wound until the healing process is complete.

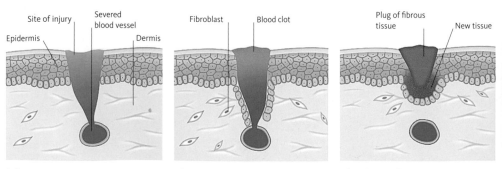

Injury
At the site of injury, platelets in the blood arrive to begin formation of a clot. Other cells are attracted to the site to help with repair.

Clotting
A clot is formed by platelets in the blood and blood-clotting protein. Tissue-forming cells migrate to the damaged area to start repair.

Plugging and scabbing
A plug of fibrous tissue is formed within the clot. The plug hardens and forms a scab that eventually drops off when skin beneath it is healed.

TYPES OF WOUND

Wounds can be classified into a number of different types, depending on the object that produces the wound—such as a knife or a bullet—and the manner in which the wound has been inflicted.

Each of these types of wounds carries specific risks associated with surrounding tissue damage and infection.

Simple laceration

This is caused by a clean surface cut from a sharp-edged object such as a razor. Blood vessels are cut straight across, so bleeding may be profuse. Structures such as tendons or nerves may be damaged.

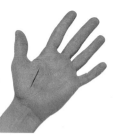

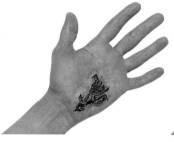

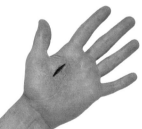

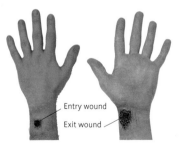

Complex Laceration

Blunt or ripping forces result in tears or lacerations. These wounds may bleed less than clean surface cuts, but there may be deep tissue damage. These lacerations are often contaminated with germs, so the risk of infection is high.

Abrasion (scrape)

This is a superficial wound in which the topmost layers of skin are scraped off, leaving a raw, tender area. Abrasions are often caused by a sliding fall or a friction burn. They can contain embedded foreign particles that may cause infection.

Contusion (bruise)

A blunt blow can rupture capillaries beneath the skin, causing blood to leak into the tissues. This process results in bruising. Extensive contusion and swelling may indicate deeper damage, such as a fracture or an internal injury.

Entry wound

Exit wound

Puncture wound

An injury such as standing on a nail or being pricked by a needle will result in a puncture wound. It has a small entry site but a deep track of internal damage. Since germs and dirt can be carried far into the body, the infection risk with this kind of wound is high.

Stab wound

This is a deep incision caused by a long or bladed instrument, usually a knife, penetrating the body. Stab wounds to the trunk must always be treated as serious because of the danger of injury to vital organs and life-threatening internal bleeding.

Gunshot wound

This type of wound is caused by a bullet or missile being driven into the body, causing serious internal injury as well as infection caused by clothing and contaminants from the air being sucked into the wound. It is important to note the number of wounds.

SHOCK

- Do not allow the casualty to eat or drink because an anesthetic may be needed. If he complains of thirst, moisten his lips with a little water.
- Do not leave the casualty unattended, unless you have to call emergency help.
- Do not warm the casualty with a hot-water bottle or other direct sources of heat, but do cover him with a blanket.
- If the casualty is in the later stages of pregnancy, help her lie down leaning toward her left side to prevent the pregnant uterus from restricting blood flow back to the heart.
- If the casualty loses consciousness, assess for normal breathing and, if absent, begin CPR with chest compressions (pp.54–87).

This is a life-threatening condition that occurs when the circulatory system fails and vital organs such as the heart and brain are deprived of oxygen. It requires immediate emergency treatment. Shock can be made worse by fear and pain. Minimize the risk of shock developing by reassuring the casualty and making him comfortable.

The most common cause of shock is severe blood loss. If this exceeds 2 pints (1.2 liters), shock will develop. This degree of blood loss may result from external bleeding. It may also be caused by: hidden bleeding from internal organs (p.116), blood escaping into a body cavity (p.116), or bleeding from damaged blood vessels due to a closed fracture (p.136 and p.138). Loss of other body fluids can also result in shock. Conditions that can cause severe fluid loss include diarrhea, vomiting, bowel obstruction, serious burns, and blood infection.

Shock may also occur when there is sufficient blood volume but the heart is unable to pump the blood around the body. This can be due to severe heart disease, heart attack, or acute heart failure (cardiogenic shock). Other causes of shock include overwhelming infection (septic shock), severe allergic reaction (anaphylactic shock), and spinal cord injury (neurogenic shock).

EFFECTS OF BLOOD OR FLUID LOSS

APPROXIMATE VOLUME LOST	EFFECTS ON THE BODY
Less than 1½ pints (0.75 liter)	■ Little or no effect; this is the quantity of blood normally taken when donating blood
1½–3¼ pints (0.75–1.5 liters)	■ Heart and respiratory rates quicken ■ Small blood vessels in nonvital areas, such as the skin, shut down to divert blood and oxygen to the vital organs, so the skin may feel cool, especially at the fingers and toes ■ Anxiety is common
3¼–4 pints (1.5–2 liters)	■ Heart and respiratory rates increase even more ■ Blood pressure drops and the brain may not receive enough oxygen, leading to increased anxiety and/or confusion ■ The pulse at the wrist may become undetectable
More than 4 pints (2 liters) (over a third of the normal volume in the average adult)	■ Heart and respiratory rates increase until the body can no longer sustain them, at which time point they decrease, a very ominous sign that often precedes death. ■ Skin may be cool and pale. ■ The casualty is likely to be unconcious

SEE ALSO Anaphylactic shock **p.223** | Internal bleeding **p.116** | Severe burns and scalds **pp.174–75** | Severe external bleeding **pp.114–15** | Spinal injury **pp.157–59** | The unconscious casualty **pp.54–87**

WHAT TO DO

1 Treat any possible cause of shock that you can detect, such as severe bleeding (pp.114–15) or serious burns (pp.174–75). Reassure the casualty.

2 Help the casualty lie down—on a rug or blanket if there is one, because this will protect him from the cold. Raise and support his legs above the level of his heart to improve blood supply to the vital organs.

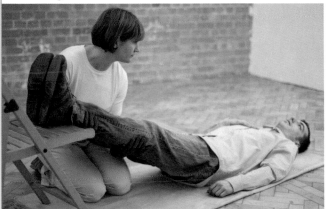

3 Call 911 for emergency help. Tell the dispatcher that you suspect shock.

4 Loosen tight clothing to reduce constriction at the neck, chest, and waist.

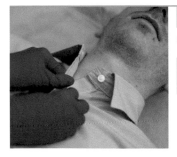

5 Keep the casualty warm by covering his body and legs with coats or blankets.

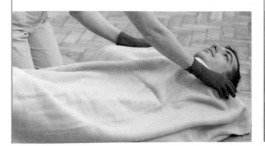

6 Monitor and record vital signs—level of response, breathing, and pulse (pp.52–53)—while waiting for help to arrive.

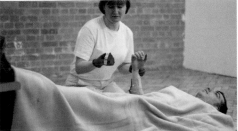

SEVERE EXTERNAL BLEEDING

YOUR AIMS

- To control bleeding
- To prevent and minimize the effects of shock
- To minimize infection
- To arrange urgent removal to the hospital

When bleeding is severe, it can be dramatic and distressing. If bleeding is not controlled, shock may develop and the casualty may lose consciousness.

Bleeding from the mouth or nose may affect breathing. When treating severe bleeding, check first whether there is an object embedded in the wound; take care not to press directly on the object. Do not let the casualty have anything to eat or drink because he may need an anesthetic later.

WHAT TO DO

1 **Remove or cut clothing** as necessary to expose the wound (p.232).

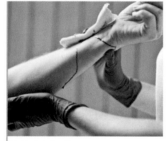

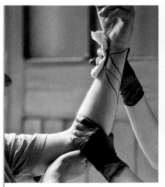

2 **Apply direct pressure** over the wound with your fingers using a sterile dressing or clean, gauze pad. If you do not have a dressing, ask the casualty to apply direct pressure himself. If there is an object in the wound, apply pressure on either side of the object (opposite).

3 **Maintain direct pressure** on the wound to control bleeding. Raise and support the injured limb above the level of the casualty's heart to reduce blood loss.

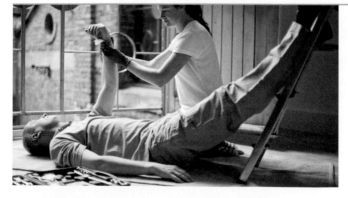

4 **Help the casualty lie down**—on a rug or blanket if there is one, because this will protect him from the cold. Since shock may develop (pp.112–13), raise and support his legs so that they are above the level of his heart. Ask a helper to **call 911 for emergency help**, and to give the dispatcher details of the site and extent of the bleeding.

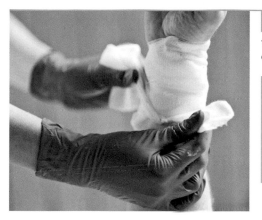

5 Secure the dressing with a bandage that is firm enough to maintain pressure, but not so tight that it impairs circulation (p.243). **Call 911 for emergency help** if this has not been done already.

6 If bleeding shows through the dressing, apply a second one on top of the first. If blood seeps through the second dressing, remove both and apply a fresh one, ensuring that pressure is applied accurately at the point of bleeding.

7 Support the injured part in a raised position with a sling and/or bandage. Check the circulation beyond the bandage every ten minutes (p.243). If the circulation is impaired, loosen the bandage and reapply.

8 Monitor and record vital signs—level of response, breathing, and pulse (pp.52–53)—while waiting for help to arrive.

SPECIAL CASE IF THERE IS AN OBJECT IN THE WOUND

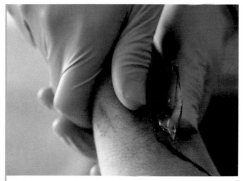

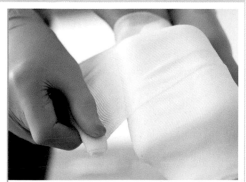

1 Control bleeding by pressing firmly on either side of the embedded object to push the edges of the wound together. Do not press directly on the object, or try to remove it. Raise the injury above the level of the heart.

3 Treat for shock (pp.112–13). **Call 911 for emergency help.** Monitor and record vital signs—level of response, breathing, and pulse (pp.52–53)—while waiting for help to arrive.

2 To protect the wound, drape a piece of gauze over the object. Build up padding on either side, then carefully bandage over the object and pads without pressing on the object (p.121). Check the circulation beyond the bandage every ten minutes (p.243). If the circulation is impaired, loosen the bandage and reapply.

INTERNAL BLEEDING

RECOGNITION

- Initially, pale, cold, clammy skin. If bleeding continues, the skin may turn blue-gray (cyanosis)
- Rapid, weak pulse
- Thirst
- Rapid, shallow breathing
- Confusion, restlessness, and irritability
- Possible collapse and unconsciousness
- Bleeding from body openings (orifices)
- In cases of violent injury, "pattern bruising"—an area of discolored skin with a shape that matches the pattern of clothes or crushing or restraining objects
- Pain
- Information from the casualty that indicates recent injury or illness

Bleeding inside body cavities may follow an injury, such as a fracture or a blow from a blunt object, but it can also occur spontaneously—for example, bleeding from a stomach ulcer. The main risk from internal bleeding is shock (pp.112–13). In addition, blood can build up around organs such as the lungs or brain and exert damaging pressure on them.

Suspect internal bleeding if a casualty develops signs of shock without obvious blood loss. Check for any bleeding from body openings such as the ear, mouth, and nose. There may also be bleeding from the urethra, vagina, or anus (below).

The signs of bleeding vary depending on the site of the blood loss (below), but the most obvious is a discharge of blood from a body opening. Blood loss from any orifice is significant and can lead to shock. In addition, bleeding from some orifices can indicate a serious underlying injury or illness. Follow treatment for shock (pp.112–13).

POSSIBLE SIGNS OF INTERNAL BLEEDING

SITE	APPEARANCE OF BLOOD	CAUSE OF BLOOD LOSS
Mouth	■ Bright red, frothy, coughed-up blood	■ Bleeding in lungs
	■ Vomited blood, red or dark reddish brown, resembling coffee grounds	■ Bleeding within digestive system
Ear	■ Fresh, bright red blood	■ Injury to inner or outer ear or perforated eardrum
	■ Thin, watery blood	■ Leakage of fluid from around brain due to head injury (skull fracture)
Nose	■ Fresh, bright red blood	■ Ruptured blood vessel in nostril
	■ Thin, watery blood	■ Leakage of fluid from around brain due to head injury (skull fracture)
Anus	■ Fresh, bright red blood	■ Hemorrhoids ■ Injury to anus or lower intestine ■ Brisk upper gastrointestinal bleeding
	■ Black, tarry stool (melena)	■ Disease or injury to intestine
Urethra	■ Red or smoky appearance to urine, occasionally containing clots	■ Bleeding from bladder, kidneys, or urethra
Vagina	■ Either fresh or dark blood	■ Menstruation ■ Miscarriage ■ Ectopic pregnancy ■ Pregnancy ■ Recent childbirth ■ Assault

IMPALEMENT

If someone has been impaled, for example by falling onto railings, never attempt to lift the casualty off the object involved because this may worsen internal injuries. Call the emergency services immediately, giving clear details about the incident. They will bring special cutting equipment with them to free the casualty.

WHAT TO DO

1 **Call 911 for emergency help.** Send a helper to make the call, if possible. Explain the situation clearly to the dispatcher, so that the right equipment will be brought.

2 **Support the casualty's body weight** until the emergency services arrive and take over. Reassure the casualty while you wait for emergency help.

CAUTION
- Do not allow the casualty to eat or drink because an anesthetic may be needed.

YOUR AIM
- To prevent further injury

AMPUTATION

A limb that has been partially or completely severed can, in many cases, be reattached by microsurgery. The operation will require a general anesthetic, so do not allow the casualty to eat or drink. It is vital to get the casualty and the amputated part to the hospital as soon as possible. Shock is possible, and needs to be treated.

WHAT TO DO

1 **Control blood loss** by applying direct pressure and raising the injured part above the casualty's heart.

2 **Place a sterile dressing** or a clean gauze pad on the wound, and secure it with a bandage. If you are trained to use a tourniquet, it may be appropriate. Treat the casualty for shock (pp.112–13).

3 **Call 911 for emergency help.** Tell the dispatcher that an amputation is involved. Monitor and record vital signs—level of response, breathing, and pulse (pp.52–53)—while waiting for help to arrive.

4 **Wrap the severed part** in plastic wrap or a plastic bag. Wrap the package in gauze or soft fabric and place it in a container full of crushed ice. Mark the container with the time of injury and the casualty's name. Give it to the emergency service personnel yourself.

CAUTION
- Do not wash the severed part.
- Do not let the severed part touch the crushed ice when packing it.
- Do not allow the casualty to eat or drink because an anesthetic may be needed.

YOUR AIMS
- To control bleeding
- To minimize the effects of shock
- To arrange urgent removal to the hospital
- To prevent deterioration of the injured part

SEE ALSO Severe external bleeding **pp.114–15** | Shock **pp.112–13**

CRUSH INJURY

YOUR AIM

- To obtain specialist medical aid urgently, taking any steps possible to treat the casualty

Traffic accidents and building site collapses are the most common causes of crush injuries. Other possible causes include explosions, earthquakes, and train crashes.

A crush injury may include a fracture, swelling, and internal bleeding. The crushing force may cause impaired circulation, resulting in numbness at or below the site of injury. You may not detect a pulse in a crushed limb.

DANGERS OF PROLONGED CRUSHING

If the casualty is trapped for any length of time, two serious complications may result. First, prolonged crushing may cause extensive damage to body tissues, especially to muscles. Once the pressure is removed, shock may develop rapidly as tissue fluid leaks into the injured area.

More dangerous, toxic substances build up in damaged muscle tissue around a crush injury. If released suddenly into the circulation, these toxins may cause the heart to experience a life-threatening rhythm disturbance first or kidney failure later. This process, called "crush syndrome," is extremely serious and can be fatal.

WHAT TO DO

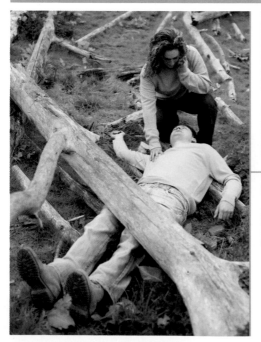

1 **If you know the casualty** has been crushed for less than 15 minutes and you can release him, do this as quickly as possible. Control external bleeding and steady and support any suspected fracture (pp.136–38). Treat the casualty for shock (pp.112–13) but do not raise his legs.

2 **If the casualty has been crushed for more** than 15 minutes, or you cannot move the cause of injury, leave him in the position found and comfort and reassure him.

3 **Call 911 for emergency help,** giving clear details of the incident to the dispatcher.

4 **Monitor and record vital signs**—level of response, breathing, and pulse (pp.52–53)—while waiting for help to arrive.

| **SEE ALSO** Fractures **pp.136–38** | Severe external bleeding **pp.114–15** | Shock **pp.112–13**

CUTS AND SCRAPES

Bleeding from small cuts and scrapes is easily controlled by pressure and elevation. An adhesive bandage is normally all that is required, and the wound will heal by itself in a few days. Medical help needs to be sought only if: bleeding does not stop; there is a foreign object embedded in the cut (p.121); there is a particular risk of infection, from a human or animal bite (p.203), or a puncture by a dirty object; or an old wound shows signs of becoming infected (p.120).

WHAT TO DO

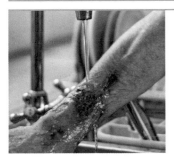

1 **If the wound is dirty,** clean it by rinsing under running water, or use alcohol-free wipes. Pat the wound dry using a gauze swab and cover it with sterile gauze.

2 **Raise and support** the injured part above the level of the heart, if possible. Avoid touching the wound.

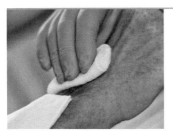

3 **Clean the area** around the wound with soap and water. Wipe away from the wound and use a clean swab for each stroke. Pat dry. Remove the wound covering and apply a sterile dressing. If there is a particular risk of infection, advise the casualty to seek medical advice.

YOUR AIMS

- To control bleeding
- To minimize the risk of infection

SPECIAL CASE TETANUS

This is a dangerous infection caused by a bacterium that lives in soil. If it enters a wound, it may multiply in the damaged tissues and release a toxin that spreads through the nervous system, causing muscle spasms, paralysis, and death. Tetanus can be prevented by immunization, which is normally given in childhood and repeated as boosters in adulthood.

BRUISING

Caused by bleeding into the skin or into tissues beneath the skin, a bruise can either develop rapidly or emerge a few days after injury. Bruising can also indicate deep injury. Elderly people and those taking anticoagulant (anticlotting) drugs, such as aspirin or warfarin, can bruise easily.

YOUR AIM

- To reduce blood flow to the injury, in order to minimize swelling

WHAT TO DO

1 **Raise and support** the injured part in a comfortable position.

2 **Place** a cold compress (p.241). over the bruise for at least ten minutes.

BLISTERS

Blisters occur when the skin is repeatedly rubbed against another surface or when it is exposed to heat. The damaged area of skin leaks tissue fluid that collects under the top layer of the skin, forming a blister.

WHAT TO DO

1 Wash the area with clean water and rinse. Gently pat the area and surrounding skin thoroughly dry with a sterile gauze pad. If it is not possible to wash the area, keep it as clean as possible.

2 Cover the blister with an adhesive dressing; make sure the pad of the bandage is larger than the blister. Ideally use a blister bandage, which has a cushioned pad that provides extra protection and comfort.

INFECTED WOUND

RECOGNITION

■ Increasing pain and soreness at the site of the wound

■ Swelling, redness, and a feeling of heat around the injury

■ Pus within, or oozing from, the wound

■ Swelling and tenderness of the glands in the neck, armpit, or groin

■ Faint red trails on the skin that lead to the glands in the neck, armpit, or groin

If infection is advanced:

■ Signs of fever, such as sweating, thirst, shivering, and lethargy

YOUR AIMS

■ To prevent further infection

■ To obtain medical advice if necessary

An open wound can become contaminated with microorganisms (germs). The germs may come from the source of the injury, from the environment, from the mouth, the fingers, or from particles of clothing embedded in a wound (as may occur in gunshot wounds). Bleeding may flush some dirt away; remaining germs may be destroyed by the white blood cells. However, if dirt or dead tissue remain in a wound, infection may spread through the body. There is also a risk of tetanus (p.119).

Any wound that does not begin to heal within 48 hours is likely to be infected. A casualty with a wound that is at high risk of infection may need treatment with antibiotics and/or tetanus immunization (p.119).

WHAT TO DO

 1 **Cover the wound with a sterile dressing** or large clean, nonstick pad, and bandage it in place.

 2 **Raise and support the injured part** with a sling and/or bandages. This helps reduce the swelling around the injury.

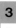 **3** **Advise the casualty to seek medical advice.** If infection is advanced (with signs of fever, such as sweating, shivering, and lethargy), take or send the casualty to the hospital.

FOREIGN OBJECT IN A WOUND

It is important to remove foreign objects, such as small pieces of glass or grit, from a wound before beginning treatment. If left in a wound, they may cause infection or delay healing. The best way to remove superficial pieces of glass or grit from the skin is to pick them out with tweezers. Alternatively, rinse loose pieces off with running water. Do not try to remove pieces that are firmly embedded in the wound because you may damage the surrounding tissue and aggravate bleeding. Instead, cover the object with a dressing and bandage and take the casualty to a healthcare provider.

CAUTION

- Ask the casualty about tetanus immunization. Seek medical advice if:
- He has a dirty wound.
- He has never been immunized.
- He is not sure he is up to date with his immunizations.

WHAT TO DO

1 Control bleeding by applying pressure on either side of the object (see p.115) and raising the area above the casualty's heart level. Drape a piece of gauze over the wound and object.

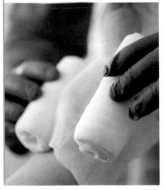

2 Build up padding on either side of the object (rolled bandages make good padding) until it is high enough for you to be able to bandage over the object without pressing it farther into the wound. Hold the padding in place until the bandaging is complete.

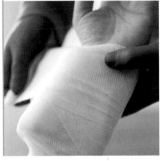

YOUR AIMS

- To control bleeding without pressing the object farther into the wound
- To minimize the risk of infection
- To arrange transportation to the hospital if necessary

3 Arrange to take or send the casualty to the hospital.

SPECIAL CASE BANDAGING AROUND A LARGER OBJECT

Never remove impaled objects, such as pencils, knives, or branches. If you cannot build padding high enough to bandage over the top of an object, drape a clean piece of gauze over it. Place padding on either side of the object, then secure it in place by bandaging above and below the object.

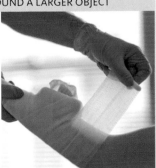

SEE ALSO Cuts and scrapes **p.119** | Embedded fishhook **p.195** | Severe external bleeding **pp.114–15** | Splinter **p.194** | 121

SCALP AND HEAD WOUNDS

YOUR AIMS

- To control bleeding
- To arrange transportation to the hospital

The scalp has many small blood vessels running close to the skin surface, so any cut can result in profuse bleeding, which often makes a scalp wound appear worse than it is.

In some cases, however, a scalp wound may form part of a more serious underlying head injury, such as a skull fracture, or may be associated with a neck injury. For these reasons, you should examine a casualty with a scalp wound very carefully, particularly if it is possible that signs of a serious head injury are being masked by alcohol or drug intoxication. If you are in any doubt, follow the treatment for head injury (p.144–45). In addition, bear in mind the possibility of a neck (spinal) injury.

WHAT TO DO

1 If there are any displaced flaps of skin at the injury site, carefully replace them over the wound. Reassure the casualty.

2 Cover the wound with a sterile dressing or a large clean, gauze pad. Apply firm, direct pressure on the pad to help control bleeding to reduce blood loss, and minimize the risk of shock.

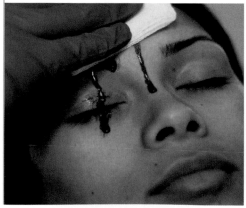

3 Keep the pad in place with a roller bandage to secure the pad and maintain pressure.

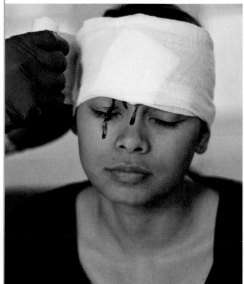

4 Help the casualty lie down with her head and shoulders slightly raised. If she feels faint or dizzy or shows any signs of shock, **call 911 for emergency help.** Monitor and record vital signs—level of response, breathing, and pulse (pp.52–53)—while waiting for help.

| **SEE ALSO** Head injury p.144–45 | Shock pp.112–13 | Spinal injury pp.157–59

EYE WOUND

The eye can be bruised or cut by direct blows or by sharp, chipped fragments of metal, grit, and glass.

All eye injuries are potentially serious because of the risk to the casualty's vision. Even superficial abrasions to the surface (cornea) of the eye can lead to scarring or infection, with the possibility of permanent deterioration of vision.

WHAT TO DO

1 Help the casualty into a half-sitting position or onto on his back, and hold his head to keep it as still as possible. Tell him to keep both eyes still because movement of the "good" eye will cause movement of the injured one, which may damage it further.

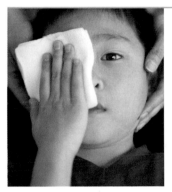

2 Give the casualty a sterile dressing or a clean, nonfluffy pad to hold over the affected eye. If it will take some time to obtain medical help, secure the pad in place with a bandage. Do not apply pressure to the injured eye.

3 Arrange to take or send the casualty to the hospital.

CAUTION
- Do not touch or attempt to remove anything that is sticking to, or embedded in, the eyeball or on the colored part (iris) of the eye. Instead, place a paper cup over the affected eye and bandage it in place.

RECOGNITION
- Pain in the eye or eyelids
- Visible wound and/or bloodshot appearance
- Partial or total loss of vision
- Leakage of blood or clear fluid from a wound

YOUR AIMS
- To prevent further damage
- To arrange transportation to the hospital

BLEEDING FROM THE EAR

This may be due to a burst (perforated) eardrum, an ear infection, a blow to the side of the head, or an explosion. Symptoms include a sharp pain, earache, deafness, and possibly dizziness. The presence of blood or blood-stained watery fluid indicates a more serious, underlying head injury (pp.144–45).

WHAT TO DO

1 Help the casualty into a half-sitting position, with his head tilted to the injured side to allow blood to drain from the ear.

2 Hold a sterile dressing or a clean, gauze pad lightly in place on the ear. Do not plug the ear. Send or take the casualty to the hospital.

CAUTION
- If you suspect a head injury (pp.144–45), support the casualty's head in the position you found him and **call 911 for emergency help.**

YOUR AIM
- To arrange transportation to the hospital.

NOSEBLEED

YOUR AIMS

- To maintain an open airway
- To control bleeding

Bleeding from the nose most commonly occurs when tiny blood vessels inside the nostrils are ruptured, either by a blow to the nose, or as a result of sneezing, picking, or blowing the nose. Nosebleeds may also occur as a result of high blood pressure and anticlotting medication.

A nosebleed can be serious if the casualty loses a lot of blood. In addition, if bleeding follows a head injury, the blood may appear thin and watery. The latter is a very serious sign because it indicates that the skull is fractured and fluid is leaking from around the brain.

WHAT TO DO

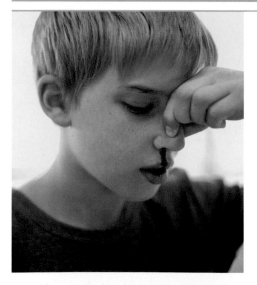

1 Tell the casualty to sit down and tilt his head forward to allow the blood to drain from the nostrils. Ask him to breathe through his mouth (this will have a calming effect) and to pinch the soft part of his nose for up to ten minutes, holding constant pressure. Reassure and help him if necessary.

2 Advise the casualty not to speak, swallow, cough, spit, or sniff since this may disturb blood clots that have formed in the nose. Give him a clean cloth or tissue to mop up any dribbling.

3 After ten minutes, tell the casualty to release the pressure. If the bleeding has not stopped, tell him to reapply the pressure for two further periods of ten minutes.

4 Once the bleeding has stopped, and with the casualty still leaning forward, clean around his nose with lukewarm water. Advise him to rest quietly for a few hours. Tell him to avoid exertion and, in particular, not to blow his nose, because this could disturb any clots.

5 If bleeding stops and then restarts, help the casualty reapply pressure.

6 If the nosebleed is severe, or if it lasts longer than 30 minutes, arrange to take or send the casualty to the hospital.

SPECIAL CASE FOR A YOUNG CHILD

A child may be worried by a nosebleed. Tell her to lean forward, and then pinch her nose for her, reassure her, and give her a bowl to spit or dribble into.

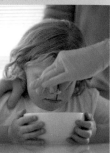

KNOCKED-OUT ADULT TOOTH

If a secondary (adult) tooth is knocked out, it should be replanted in its socket as soon as possible. Gently rinse off any dirt before replacing it in the socket. If this is not possible, ask the casualty to keep the tooth inside his cheek or under his tongue if he feels able to do this without swallowing the tooth. Alternatively, place it in a small container of milk to prevent it from drying out.

CAUTION

- Do not clean off any fleshy debris—you may damage the tissues, reducing the chance of reimplantation.

WHAT TO DO

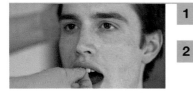

1 Gently push the tooth into the socket. Then press a gauze pad between the bottom and top teeth to help keep the tooth in place.

2 Ask the casualty to hold the tooth firmly in place. Send him to a dentist or the hospital.

BLEEDING FROM THE MOUTH

Cuts to the tongue, lips, or lining of the mouth range from minor injuries to more serious wounds. The cause is usually the casualty's own teeth or dental extraction. Bleeding from the mouth may be profuse and can be alarming. In addition, there is a danger that blood may be inhaled into the lungs, causing problems with breathing.

CAUTION

- If the wound is large, or bleeding lasts longer than 30 minutes or restarts, seek medical or dental advice.

WHAT TO DO

1 Ask the casualty to sit down, with her head forward and tilted slightly to the injured side, to allow blood to drain from her mouth. Place a sterile gauze pad over the wound. Ask the casualty to squeeze the pad between finger and thumb and press on the wound for ten minutes.

2 If bleeding persists, replace the pad. Tell the casualty to let the blood dribble out; if she swallows it, it may induce vomiting. Do not wash the mouth out because this may disturb a clot. Advise her to avoid drinking anything hot for 12 hours.

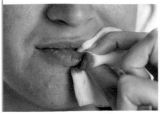

YOUR AIMS

- To control bleeding
- To safeguard the airway by preventing any inhalation of blood

SPECIAL CASE
BLEEDING SOCKET

To control bleeding from a tooth socket, roll a gauze pad or tea bag thick enough to keep the casualty's teeth from meeting, place it across the empty socket, and tell him to bite down on it.

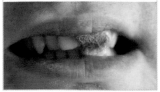

FINGER WOUND

YOUR AIMS

- To control bleeding
- To assess whether or not the wound needs a medical assessment

Injuries to the fingers are common and can vary from small cuts and scrapes to wounds with underlying damage to bones, tendons, and ligaments. Injuries to the nails are the most common. All finger wounds need good management because the hand is a finely coordinated part of the body that must function correctly for many everyday activities.

A cut to a finger may go through the skin only or it can cut through blood vessels, nerves, and tendons that lie just under the skin. There will be bleeding, which can be profuse, and possibly bruising, deformity, or loss of movement or sensation if the underlying structures are damaged.

WHAT TO DO

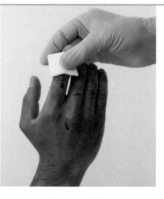

1 If the wound to the finger breaks the skin, it should be cleaned with soap and water like any other abrasion.

2 Press a sterile dressing or clean gauze pad on the wound and apply direct pressure to control bleeding.

3 Raise and support the injured hand and maintain pressure on the wound until the bleeding stops.

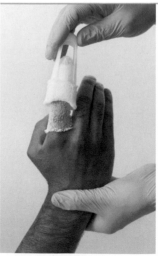

4 When the bleeding has stopped, cover the wound to protect it. Use an adhesive dressing or for a larger wound apply a dressing pad, secured with a tubular gauze bandage. If there is a fracture or dislocation, the finger should be splinted.

5 Seek medical help if necessary. If you need to take the casualty to the hospital, support the injured arm in an elevation sling (p.252).

WOUND TO THE PALM

The palm of the hand has a good blood supply, which is why a wound there may cause profuse bleeding. A deep wound to the palm may sever tendons and nerves in the hand and result in loss of feeling or movement in the fingers.

Bandaging the fist can be an effective way to control bleeding. If, however, a casualty has a foreign object embedded in a palm wound, it will be impossible to clench the fist. In such cases, control the bleeding and bandage the injury using the method described on p.121.

YOUR AIMS

- To control bleeding and minimize the risk of shock
- To minimize the risk of infection
- To arrange transportation to the hospital

WHAT TO DO

1 If the wound to the palm breaks the skin, it should be cleaned with soap and water.

2 Press a sterile dressing or clean pad firmly into the palm, and ask the casualty to clench his fist over it or to grasp his fist with his other hand.

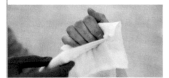

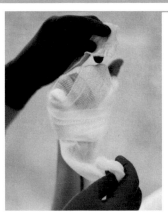

3 **Raise and support the hand.** Bandage the casualty's fingers so that they are clenched over the pad; leave the thumb free so that you can check circulation. Tie the ends of the bandage over the top of the fingers to help maintain pressure.

4 **Support the arm** in an elevation sling (p.252). Arrange to take or send him to the hospital.

WOUND AT A JOINT CREASE

Large blood vessels pass across the inside of the elbow and back of the knee. If severed, these vessels will bleed profusely. The steps given below help control bleeding and shock. Take care to ensure that there is adequate circulation to the part of the limb beyond the bandage.

YOUR AIMS

- To control bleeding
- To prevent and minimize the effects of shock
- To arrange transportation to the hospital

WHAT TO DO

1 **Firmly press a sterile dressing** or clean gauze pad on the injury. If the casualty is alone and must apply pressure himself, it may help to bend the joint as far as it will go, holding the pad firmly in place.

2 Raise and support the limb. If possible, help the casualty lie down with his legs raised and supported. If you are unable to control the bleeding and you are trained to use a tourniquet, it may be appropriate to do so.

3 Arrange to take or send him to the hospital. **Every ten minutes,** check the circulation (p.243) in the lower part of the limb. If there is no pulse, loosen the dressing a bit. If active bleeding recurs, tighten it.

ABDOMINAL WOUND

YOUR AIMS

- To minimize shock
- To arrange urgent removal to the hospital

A stab wound, gunshot, or crush injury to the abdomen may cause a serious wound. Organs and large blood vessels can be punctured, lacerated, or ruptured. There may be external bleeding, protruding abdominal contents, and internal bleeding and injury. External bleeding and wounds can be treated as below.

WHAT TO DO

1 Help the casualty lie down on a firm surface, on a blanket if available. Loosen any tight clothing, such as a belt or a shirt.

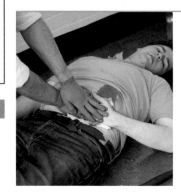

2 Cover wound with a sterile dressing and hold it firmly; the casualty may be able to help. Raise and support the casualty's knees to ease strain on injury.

3 Call 911 for emergency help. Treat the casualty for shock (pp.112–13). Monitor and record vital signs—breathing, pulse, and level of response—(pp.52–53) while waiting for help to arrive.

VAGINAL BLEEDING

YOUR AIMS

- To make the woman comfortable and reassure her
- To arrange removal to the hospital if necessary

Be sensitive to the woman's feelings. The bleeding is possibly menstrual bleeding, but it can also indicate a more serious condition such as miscarriage, pregnancy including ruptured ectopic pregnancy, recent termination of pregnancy, childbirth, or injury as a result of sexual assault. If the bleeding is severe, shock may develop.

If a woman has been sexually assaulted, it is vital to preserve the evidence if possible. Gently advise her to refrain from washing or using the toilet until a forensic examination has been performed. If she wishes to remove clothing, keep it intact in a clean paper bag if possible. Be aware that she may feel vulnerable and may prefer to be treated by a woman.

1 Allow the woman privacy and give her a sanitary napkin. Make her comfortable in whichever position she prefers.

2 If she has menstrual period pains, she may take the recommended dose of acetaminophen or ibuprofen.

BLEEDING VARICOSE VEIN

Veins contain one-way valves that keep the blood flowing toward the heart. If these valves fail, blood collects (pools) behind them and makes the veins swell. This problem, called varicose veins, usually develops in the legs.

A varicose vein has taut, thin walls and is often raised, typically producing knobbly skin over the affected area. The vein can be burst by a gentle knock, and this may result in profuse bleeding. Shock will quickly develop if bleeding is not controlled.

YOUR AIMS

■ To control bleeding
■ To prevent and minimize shock
■ To arrange urgent removal to the hospital

WHAT TO DO

1 **Help the casualty lie down** on his back. Raise and support the injured leg as high as possible immediately, because this reduces the amount of bleeding.

2 **Rest the injured leg** on your shoulder or on a chair. Apply firm, direct pressure on the injury, using a sterile dressing, or a clean gauze pad, until the blood loss is under control. If necessary, carefully cut away clothing to expose the site of the bleeding.

3 **Remove garments such as girdles** or pantyhose because these may cause the bleeding to continue.

4 **Keeping the leg raised,** put another large, soft pad over the dressing. Bandage it firmly enough to exert even pressure, but not so tightly that the circulation in the limb is impaired.

5 **Call 911 for emergency help.** Keep the injured leg raised and supported until the ambulance arrives. Monitor and record vital signs—level of response, breathing, and pulse (pp.52–53)—regularly until help arrives. In addition, check the circulation in the limb beyond the bandage (p.243) every ten minutes.

7

The skeleton is the supporting framework around which the body is constructed. It is jointed in many places, and muscles attached to the bones enable us to move. Most of our movements are controlled at will and coordinated by impulses that travel from the brain via the nerves to every muscle and joint in the body.

It is difficult for a first aider to distinguish between different bone, joint, and muscle injuries, so this chapter begins with an overview of how bones, muscles, and joints function and how injuries affect them. First aid treatments for most injuries, from serious fractures to sprains, strains, and dislocations, are included here in this section.

First aid for head and spinal injuries is also covered in the chapter. There is anatomical information about the nervous system that explains how these injuries can be made worse by potential damage to the damage and spinal cord.

AIMS AND OBJECTIVES

- To assess the casualty's condition quickly and calmly
- To support the injured part of the body
- To minimize shock
- To **call 911 for emergency help** if you suspect a serious injury
- To comfort and reassure the casualty
- To be aware of your own needs

BONE, JOINT, AND MUSCLE INJURIES

THE SKELETON

The body is built on a framework of bones called the skeleton. This structure supports the muscles, blood vessels, and nerves of the body. Many bones of the skeleton also protect important organs such as the brain and heart. At many points on the skeleton, bones articulate with each other by means of joints. These are supported by ligaments and moved by muscles that are attached to the bones by tendons.

The skeleton
There are 206 bones in the adult human skeleton, providing a protective framework for the body. The skull, spine, and rib cage protect vital body structures; the pelvis supports the abdominal organs; and the bones and joints of the arms and legs enable the body to move.

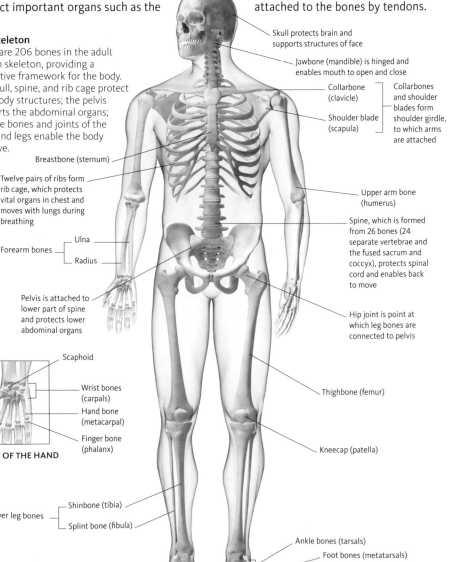

Skull protects brain and supports structures of face

Jawbone (mandible) is hinged and enables mouth to open and close

Collarbone (clavicle)

Shoulder blade (scapula)

Collarbones and shoulder blades form shoulder girdle, to which arms are attached

Breastbone (sternum)

Twelve pairs of ribs form rib cage, which protects vital organs in chest and moves with lungs during breathing

Forearm bones — Ulna
— Radius

Upper arm bone (humerus)

Spine, which is formed from 26 bones (24 separate vertebrae and the fused sacrum and coccyx), protects spinal cord and enables back to move

Pelvis is attached to lower part of spine and protects lower abdominal organs

Hip joint is point at which leg bones are connected to pelvis

Scaphoid

Wrist bones (carpals)

Hand bone (metacarpal)

Finger bone (phalanx)

BONES OF THE HAND

Thighbone (femur)

Kneecap (patella)

Lower leg bones — Shinbone (tibia)
— Splint bone (fibula)

Ankle bones (tarsals)

Foot bones (metatarsals)

THE SPINE

Also known as the backbone, the spine has a number of functions. It supports the head, makes the upper body flexible, helps support the body's weight, and protects the spinal cord (p.157). The spine is a column made up of 26 bones called vertebrae, which are connected by joints. Between individual vertebrae are disks of fibrous tissue, known as intervertebral disks, which help make the spine flexible and cushion it from jolts. Muscles and ligaments that are attached to the vertebrae help stabilize the spine and control the movements of the back.

Spinal column
The vertebrae form five groups: the cervical vertebrae support the head and neck; the thoracic vertebrae form an anchor for the ribs; the lumbar vertebrae help support the body's weight and give stability; the sacrum supports the pelvis; and the coccyx forms the end of the spine.

Structures that make the spine flexible
The joints connecting the vertebrae, and the disks between the vertebrae, allow the spine to move. There is only limited movement between adjacent vertebrae, but together the vertebrae, disks, and ligaments allow a range of movements in the spine as a whole.

Cervical spine
(7 bones)

Thoracic spine
(12 bones)

Lumbar spine
(5 bones)

Sacrum
(5 fused bones)

Coccyx
(4 fused bones)

Intervertebral disk

Projection provides an anchor for ligaments and muscles

Ligaments between vertebrae help control movement of spine

Vertebra

PORTION OF SPINE

Gelatinous core

Fibrous covering

SECTION OF DISK

THE SKULL

This bony structure protects the brain and the top of the spinal cord. It also supports the eyes and other facial structures. The skull is made up of several bones, most of which are fused at joints called sutures. Within the bone are air spaces (sinuses), which lighten the skull. The bones covering the brain form a dome called the cranium. Several other bones form the eye sockets, nose, cheeks, and jaw.

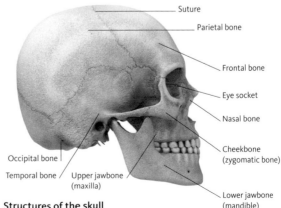

Suture

Parietal bone

Frontal bone

Eye socket

Nasal bone

Cheekbone
(zygomatic bone)

Occipital bone

Temporal bone

Upper jawbone
(maxilla)

Lower jawbone
(mandible)

Structures of the skull
This illustration shows the cranium and the main bones of the face. The jawbone is the only bone in the skull that moves significantly.

133

BONES, MUSCLES, AND JOINTS

Bone is a living tissue containing calcium and phosphorus—minerals that make it hard, rigid, and strong. From birth to early adulthood, bones grow by laying down calcium on the outside. They are also able to generate new tissue after injury. Age and certain diseases can weaken bones, making them brittle and susceptible to breaking or crumbling, either under stress or spontaneously. Inherited problems, or bone disorders such as rickets, cancer, and infections, can cause bones to become distorted and weakened. Damage to the bones during adolescence can shorten a bone or impair movement. In older people, a disorder called osteoporosis can cause the bones to lose density, making them brittle and prone to breaking.

Parts of a bone
Each bone is covered by a membrane (periosteum), which contains nerves and blood vessels. Under this membrane is a layer of compact, dense bone; at the core is spongy bone. In some bones, there is a cavity at the center containing soft tissue called bone marrow.

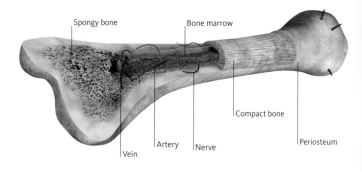

Spongy bone
Bone marrow
Compact bone
Periosteum
Nerve
Artery
Vein

THE MUSCLES

Muscles cause various parts of the body to move. Skeletal (voluntary) muscles control movement and posture. They are attached to bones by bands of strong, fibrous tissue (tendons), and many operate in groups. As one group of muscles contracts, its paired group relaxes. Involuntary muscles operate the internal organs, such as the heart, and work constantly, even while we are asleep. They are controlled by the autonomic nervous system (p.143).

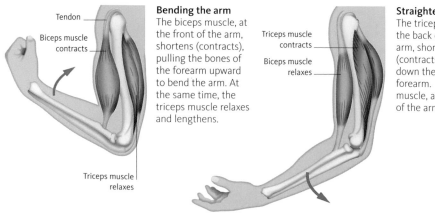

Tendon
Biceps muscle contracts
Triceps muscle relaxes

Bending the arm
The biceps muscle, at the front of the arm, shortens (contracts), pulling the bones of the forearm upward to bend the arm. At the same time, the triceps muscle relaxes and lengthens.

Triceps muscle contracts
Biceps muscle relaxes

Straightening the arm
The triceps muscle, at the back of the upper arm, shortens (contracts) to pull down the bones of the forearm. The biceps muscle, at the front of the arm, relaxes.

THE JOINTS

A joint is where one bone meets another. In a few joints (immovable joints), the bone edges fit together or are fused. Immovable joints are found in the skull and pelvis. Most joints are movable, and the bone ends are joined by fibrous tissue called ligaments, which form a capsule around the joint. The capsule lining (synovial membrane) produces fluid to lubricate the joint; the ends of the bones are also protected by smooth cartilage. Muscles that move the joint are attached to the bones by tendons. The degree and type of movement depends on the way the ends of the bones fit together, the strength of the ligaments, and the arrangement of muscles.

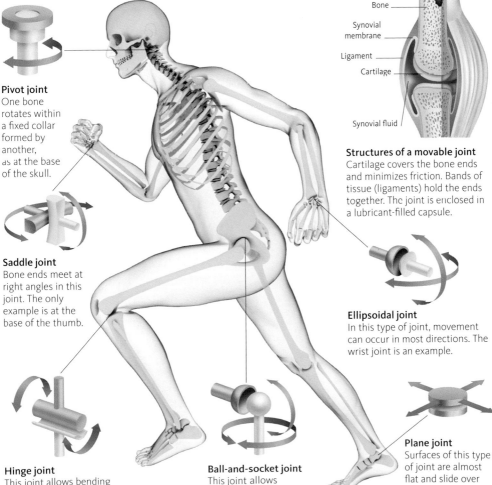

Bone
Synovial membrane
Ligament
Cartilage
Synovial fluid

Pivot joint
One bone rotates within a fixed collar formed by another, as at the base of the skull.

Structures of a movable joint
Cartilage covers the bone ends and minimizes friction. Bands of tissue (ligaments) hold the ends together. The joint is enclosed in a lubricant-filled capsule.

Saddle joint
Bone ends meet at right angles in this joint. The only example is at the base of the thumb.

Ellipsoidal joint
In this type of joint, movement can occur in most directions. The wrist joint is an example.

Hinge joint
This joint allows bending and straightening in only one plane, as in the knees and elbows.

Ball-and-socket joint
This joint allows movement in all directions. Examples are the hip and shoulder.

Plane joint
Surfaces of this type of joint are almost flat and slide over each other. This joint is found in the wrist and foot.

135

FRACTURES

There may be:

- Deformity, swelling, and bruising at the fracture site
- Pain and/or difficulty in moving the area
- Shortening, bending, or twisting of a limb
- Coarse grating (crepitus) of the bone ends that can be heard or felt (by casualty). Do not try to seek this.
- Signs of shock, especially if the thighbone or pelvis are fractured
- Difficulty in moving a limb normally or at all (for example, inability to walk)
- A wound, possibly with bone ends protruding (Treating an open fracture, p.138)

- To prevent movement at the injury site
- To arrange transportation to the hospital, with comfortable support during transit

A break or crack in a bone is called a fracture. Considerable force is needed to break a bone, unless it is diseased or old. However, bones that are still growing are supple and may split, bend, or crack like a twig. A bone may break at the point where a heavy blow is received. Fractures may also result from a twist or a wrench (indirect force).

OPEN AND CLOSED FRACTURES

In an open fracture, one of the broken bone ends may pierce the skin surface, or there may be a wound at the fracture site. An open fracture carries a high risk of becoming infected.

In a closed fracture, the skin above the fracture is intact. However, bones may be displaced (unstable), causing internal bleeding and the casualty may develop shock (pp.112–13).

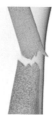

Open fracture
Bone is exposed at the surface where it breaks the skin. The casualty may suffer bleeding and shock. Infection is a risk.

Closed fracture
The skin is not broken, although the bone ends may damage nearby tissues and blood vessels. Internal bleeding is a risk.

STABLE AND UNSTABLE FRACTURES

A stable fracture occurs when the broken bone ends do not move because they are not completely broken or they are impacted. Such injuries are common at the wrist, shoulder, ankle, and hip. Usually, these fractures can be gently handled without further damage.

In an unstable fracture, the broken bone ends can easily move. There is a risk that they may damage blood vessels, nerves, and organs around the injury. Unstable injuries can occur if the bone is broken or the ligaments are torn (ruptured). They should be handled carefully to prevent further damage.

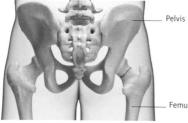

Pelvis

Femur

Stable fracture
Although the bone is fractured, the ends of the injury remain in place. The risk of bleeding or further damage is minimal.

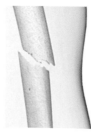

Unstable fracture
In this type of fracture, the broken bone ends can easily be displaced by movement or muscle contraction.

WHAT TO DO FOR A CLOSED FRACTURE

1 **Advise the casualty to keep still.** Support the joints above and below the injury with your hands until it is immobilized with a sling or bandages, in the position in which it is found.

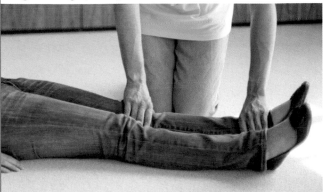

2 **Place padding around the injury** for extra support. Take or send the casualty to the hospital; a casualty with an arm injury may be transported by car; **call 911 for emergency help** for a leg injury.

3 **For firmer support** and/or if removal to the hospital is likely to be delayed, secure the injured part to an unaffected part of the body. For upper limb fractures, immobilize the arm with a sling (pp.251–52). For lower limb fractures, move the uninjured leg to the injured one and secure with broad-fold bandages (p.249). Always tie knots on the uninjured side.

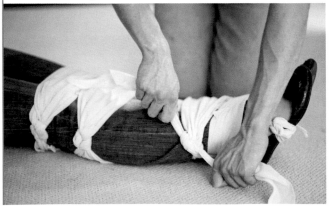

4 **Treat for shock if necessary** (pp.112–13) . Do not raise an injured leg. Elevate an uninjured limb if shock is present. Monitor and record vital signs (pp.52–53) while waiting for help. Check the circulation beyond a sling or bandage (p.243) every ten minutes. If the circulation is impaired, loosen the bandages.

‹‹ FRACTURES

CAUTION

- Do not move the casualty until the injured part is secured and supported, unless he is in immediate danger.
- Do not allow the casualty to eat or drink because an anesthetic may be needed.
- Do not press directly on a protruding bone end.

YOUR AIMS

- To prevent blood loss, movement, and infection at the site of injury
- To arrange removal to the hospital, with comfortable support

SPECIAL CASE
PROTRUDING BONE

If a bone end is protruding, build up pads of clean, soft, nonfluffy material around the bone, until you can bandage over it without pressing on the injury.

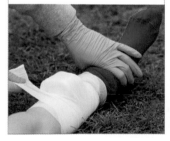

WHAT TO DO FOR AN OPEN FRACTURE

1 Cover the wound with a sterile dressing or large, clean, gauze pad. Apply pressure around the injury to control bleeding (pp.114–15); be careful not to press on a protruding bone.

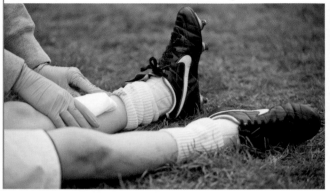

2 Carefully place a sterile wound dressing or more clean padding over and around the dressing.

3 Secure the dressing and padding with a bandage. Bandage firmly, but not so tightly that it impairs the circulation beyond the bandage.

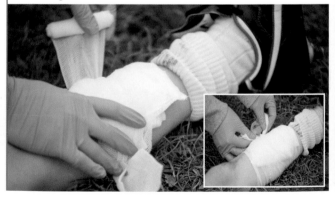

4 Immobilize the injured part as for a closed fracture (p.137), and arrange to transport the casualty to the hospital.

5 Treat the casualty for shock (pp.112–13) if necessary. Do not raise the injured leg. Monitor and record vital signs—level of response, breathing, and pulse (pp.52–53)—while waiting for help to arrive. Check the circulation beyond the bandage (p.243) every ten minutes. If the circulation is impaired, loosen the bandages.

DISLOCATED JOINT

This is a joint injury in which the bones are partially or completely pulled out of their normal position. Dislocation can be caused by a strong force wrenching the bone into an abnormal position, or by violent muscle contraction. This very painful injury most often affects the shoulder, knee, jaw, or joints in the thumbs or fingers. Dislocations may be associated with torn ligaments (pp.140–41), or with damage to the synovial membrane that lines the joint capsule (p.135).

Joint dislocation can have serious consequences. If vertebrae are dislocated, the spinal cord can be damaged. Dislocation of the shoulder or hip may damage the large nerves that supply the limbs and result in partial paralysis. A dislocation of any joint may also fracture the bones involved. It is difficult to distinguish a dislocation from a closed fracture (p.136). If you are in any doubt, treat the injury as a fracture.

CAUTION

- Do not try to replace a dislocated bone into its socket because this may cause further injury.
- Do not move the casualty until the injured part is secured and supported, unless she is in immediate danger.
- For a hand or arm injury remove bracelets, rings, and watches in case of swelling.
- Do not allow the casualty to eat or drink because an anesthetic may be needed.

RECOGNITION

There may be:
- "Sickening," severe pain
- Inability to move the joint
- Swelling and bruising around the affected joint
- Shortening, bending or deformity of the area

WHAT TO DO

1 If, for example, the casualty has a dislocated shoulder, advise the casualty to keep still. Help him support the injured arm in the position he finds most comfortable.

2 Immobilize the injured arm with a sling (p.251).

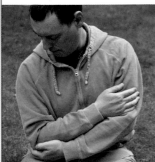
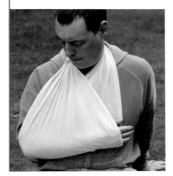

YOUR AIMS

- To prevent movement at the injury site.
- To arrange removal to the hospital, with comfortable support.

3 For extra support for an injured arm, secure the limb to the chest by tying a broad-fold bandage (p.249) around the chest and the sling.

4 Arrange to take or send the casualty to the hospital. Treat for shock if necessary. Monitor and record vital signs—level of response, breathing, and pulse—(pp.52–53) while waiting for help.

5 Check the circulation beyond the bandages (p.243) every ten minutes.

STRAINS AND SPRAINS

The softer structures around bones and joints—the ligaments, muscles, and tendons—can be injured in several ways. Injuries to these soft tissues are commonly called strains and sprains. They occur when the tissues are overstretched and partially or completely torn (ruptured) by violent or sudden movements. For this reason, strains and sprains are frequently associated with sports.

Strains and sprains should be treated initially by the "RICE" procedure:
R—**Rest** the injured part;
I—Apply **Ice** pack or a cold pad;
C—Provide comfortable support with mild **Compression** from an elastic bandage;
E—**Elevate** the injured part.
This procedure may be sufficient to relieve the symptoms, but if you are in any doubt, treat it as a fracture (pp.136–38).

MUSCLE AND TENDON INJURY

Muscles and tendons may be strained, ruptured, or bruised. A strain occurs when the muscle is overstretched; it may be partially torn, often at the junction between the muscle and the tendon that joins it to a bone. In a rupture, a muscle or tendon is torn completely; this may occur in the main bulk of the muscle or in the tendon. Deep bruising can be extensive in parts of the body where there is a large bulk of muscle. Injuries in these areas are usually accompanied by bleeding into the surrounding tissues, which can lead to pain, swelling, and bruising.

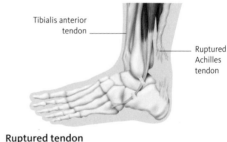

Normal muscle fibers

Torn muscle fibers produce localized pain and swelling

Tibialis anterior tendon

Ruptured Achilles tendon

Muscle tears
Vigorous movements may cause muscle fibers, such as the hamstring in the leg, to tear. Muscle tears can cause severe pain and swelling.

Ruptured tendon
The Achilles tendon attaches the calf muscle to the heel bone. It can snap after sudden exertion and may need surgery and immobilization.

LIGAMENT INJURY

One common ligament injury is a sprain. This is the stretching or tearing of a ligament at or near a joint. It is often due to a sudden or unexpected wrenching motion that pulls the bones in the joint too far apart, tearing the surrounding tissues.

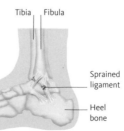

Tibia   Fibula

Sprained ligament

Heel bone

Sprained ankle
This is due to overstretching or tearing of one or more ligaments—the fibrous cords that connect bones at a joint. In this example, one of the ligaments in the ankle is partially torn.

WHAT TO DO

1 Help the casualty sit or lie down. Support the injured part in a comfortable position, preferably raised.

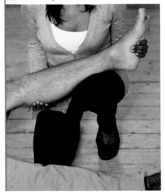

2 Cool the area by applying a cold compress, such as an ice pack in a towel (p.241), to the injury. This helps reduce swelling, bruising, and pain.

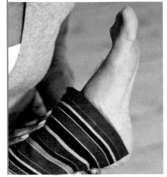

RECOGNITION

There may be:

- Pain and tenderness
- Difficulty in moving the injured part, especially if it is a joint
- Swelling and bruising in the area

YOUR AIMS

- To reduce swelling and pain
- To obtain medical help if necessary

3 Apply comfortable support to the injured part. Leave the cold compress in place or wrap an elastic bandage around the area. Secure it with a support bandage that extends to the next joint; for an ankle injury, the bandage should extend from the base of the toes to below the knee.

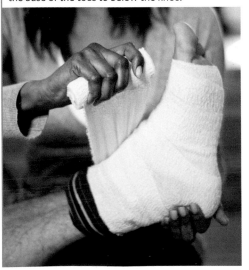

4 Support the injured part in a raised position to help minimize bruising and swelling in the area. Check the circulation beyond the bandages (p.243) every ten minutes. If the circulation is impaired, loosen the bandages.

5 If the pain is severe, or the casualty is unable to use the injured part, arrange to take or send him to the hospital. Otherwise, advise the casualty to rest the injury and to seek medical advice if necessary.

THE NERVOUS SYSTEM

The nervous system is the body's information-gathering, storage, and control system. It consists of a central processing unit—the brain—and a network of nerve cells and fibers.

There are two main parts to the nervous system: the central nervous system, consisting of the brain and spinal cord, and the peripheral nervous system, which consists of all the nerves that connect the brain and the spinal cord to the rest of the body. In addition, the autonomic (involuntary) nervous system controls body functions such as digestion, heart rate, and breathing. The central nervous system receives and analyzes information from all parts of the body. The nerves carry messages, in the form of high-speed electrical impulses, between the brain and the rest of the nervous system.

Brain

Cranial nerves (12 pairs) extend directly from the underside of the brain; most serve the head, face, neck, and shoulders

Vagus nerve, longest of the cranial nerves, serves organs in chest and abdomen; it controls the heart rate

Radial nerve controls muscles that straighten elbow and fingers

Sciatic nerve serves hip and hamstring muscles

Tibial nerve serves calf muscles

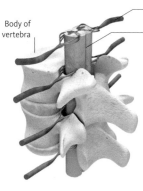

Body of vertebra

Spinal nerve

Spinal cord

Spinal cord protection
The spinal cord is protected by the vertebral column. Nerves from the spinal cord emerge between vertebrae.

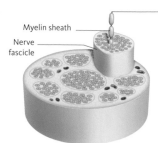

Nerve fiber

Myelin sheath

Nerve fascicle

Cross section through a nerve
Each nerve is made up of bundles of nerve fibers (fascicles). A fatty substance (myelin) surrounds and insulates larger nerve fibers.

Structure of the nervous system
The system consists of the brain, spinal cord, and a network of nerves that carry electrical impulses between the brain and the body.

CENTRAL NERVOUS SYSTEM

Together the brain and spinal cord make up the central nervous system (CNS). This system contains billions of interconnected nerve cells (neurons) and is enclosed by three membranes called meninges. A clear fluid called cerebrospinal fluid flows around the brain and spinal cord. It functions as a shock absorber, provides oxygen and nutrients, and removes waste products.

The brain has three main structures: the cerebrum, which is concerned with thought, sensation, and conscious movement; the cerebellum, which coordinates movement, balance, and posture; and the brain stem, which controls basic functions such as breathing. The main function of the spinal cord is to convey signals between the brain and the peripheral nervous system (below).

Cerebrum

Brain stem

Meninges (membranes) surround brain and spinal cord

Cerebrospinal fluid

Skull

Cerebellum

Vertebral column protects delicate spinal cord

Spinal cord extends from brain stem to lower end of spine

Structure of the brain
The brain is enclosed within the skull. It has three main parts: the cerebrum, which has an outer layer called the cortex; the cerebellum; and the brain stem.

PERIPHERAL NERVOUS SYSTEM

This part of the nervous system consists of two sets of paired nerves—the cranial and spinal nerves—connecting the CNS to the body. The cranial nerves emerge in 12 pairs from the underside of the brain. The 31 pairs of spinal nerves branch off at intervals from the spinal cord, passing into the rest of the body. Nerves comprise bundles of nerve fibers that can relay both incoming (sensory) and outgoing (motor) signals.

AUTONOMIC NERVOUS SYSTEM

Some of the cranial nerves, and several small spinal nerves, work as the autonomic nervous system. This system is concerned with vital body functions such as heart rate and breathing. The system's two parts, the sympathetic and parasympathetic systems, counterbalance each other. The sympathetic system prepares the body for action by releasing hormones that raise the heart rate and reduce the blood flow to the skin and intestines. The parasympathetic system releases hormones with a calming effect.

HEAD INJURY

ASSESSING THE LEVEL OF CONSCIOUSNESS

Assess a casualty's level of consciousness using the AVPU scale. Check the casualty at regular intervals. Make a note of your findings at each assessment, paying particular attention to any change—the casualty's condition may improve or deteriorate while you are looking after him.

A—Is the casualty **Alert**? Are his eyes open and does he respond to questions?

V—Does the casualty respond to **Voice**? Can he answer simple questions and obey commands?

P—Does the casualty respond to **Pain**? Does he move or open his eyes if pinched?

U—Is he **Unresponsive** to any stimulus?

Head injuries are common. They are potentially serious because they can lead to damage to the brain. There may also be injuries to the spine in the neck, scalp wounds and/or a skull fracture.

If a casualty has sustained a minor injury such as a bruise or scalp wound, he is likely to be fully conscious. If he has suffered a more serious blow to the head, such as in a sporting impact, consciousness may be temporarily impaired.

The brain lies inside the skull, cushioned by fluid and can therefore be shaken by a blow to the head. This is called concussion and it often produces a temporary loss of consciousness. Complications from concussion may affect thinking, language, or emotions, and may lead to problems with communication and memory, and cause personality changes, depression, and early-onset dementia.

If a casualty has suffered a severe blow to his head, this may cause bleeding or swelling inside the skull that can press on the brain (compression). This is a serious condition. The pressure can rise immediately after the impact or it may develop a few hours or even days later. The severity of the head injury is related to the mechanism of injury and its impact on the head. A serious head injury is likely after a high speed motor collision or a fall from a height.

Causes of head injury

The brain can be literally "shaken" inside the skull with concussion (below). Injury that results in bleeding can cause pressure to build up inside the skull and damage the tissues of the brain (below right).

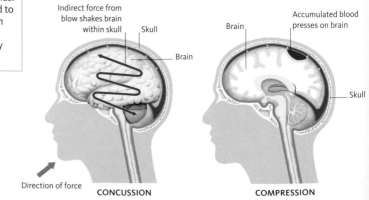

Indirect force from blow shakes brain within skull — Skull — Brain

Direction of force

CONCUSSION

Brain — Accumulated blood presses on brain — Skull

COMPRESSION

WHAT TO DO

1 Sit the casualty down and give him a cold compress to hold against the injury. Carry out an assessment of the casualty's level of consciousness using the AVPU scale (opposite). Treat any scalp wounds by applying direct pressure to the wound (p.122).

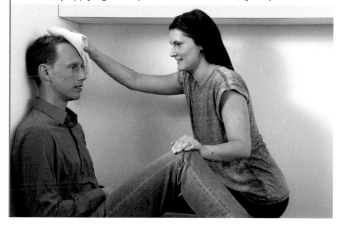

2 Regularly monitor and record vital signs—breathing, pulse and level of response (pp.52–53). Watch especially for changes in his level of response.

3 When the casualty has recovered, ask a responsible person to look after him.

4 If a casualty's injury is the result of a sporting accident, do not allow him to return to the sport until he has been fully assessed by a medical practitioner.

5 Advise the casualty to seek medical help or arrange transportation to a hospital if he develops signs and symptoms of a worsening head injury (see CAUTION, opposite, and YOUR AIMS, above), or if ANY of the following apply:
He is over 65 years of age
He has had previous brain surgery
He is taking anticoagulant (anticlotting) medication
The head injury is accompanied by drug or alcohol intoxication
There is no responsible person to look after him

RECOGNITION

There may be:
- Brief period of impaired consciousness
- Scalp wound
- Dizziness or nausea
- Loss of memory of events at the time of, or immediately preceding the injury
- Mild generalized headache
- Confusion

For severe head injury there may also be:
- History of a severe blow to the head
- Deteriorating level of response
- Loss of consciousness
- Leakage of blood or blood-stained watery fluid from the ears or nose
- Unequal pupil size

YOUR AIMS

- To place the casualty in the care of a responsible person
- To obtain medical help if the head injury is associated with loss of consciousness, confusion, or any other alteration in consciousness; if it is associated with motor or sensory defects, or persistant vomiting

SPECIAL CASE SEVERE HEAD INJURY

Call 911 for emergency help—tell the dispatcher that you suspect head injury. Maintain an open and clear airway. Do this in the position the casualty was found—try not to move him because of the additional risk of spinal injury (pp.158–59). If this is not possible, use the jaw thrust method to open the airway (p.159). Regularly monitor and record vital signs—breathing, pulse, and level of response (pp.52–53)—while waiting for help to arrive. Watch especially for changes in his level of response.

SEE ALSO Facial injury p.146 | Scalp and head wounds p.122 | The unconscious casualty pp.54–87

FACIAL INJURY

RECOGNITION

There may be:

- Pain around affected area if the jaw is affected, difficulty speaking, chewing, or swallowing
- Difficulty breathing
- Swelling and distortion of the face
- Bruising and/or a black eye
- Clear fluid or watery blood from the nose or ear

YOUR AIMS

- To keep the airway open
- To minimize pain and swelling
- To arrange urgent removal to the hospital

Fractures of facial bones are usually due to hard impacts. Serious facial fractures may appear frightening. There may be distortion of the eye sockets, general swelling and bruising, as well as bleeding from displaced tissues or from the nose and mouth. The main danger with any facial fracture is that blood, saliva or swollen tissue may obstruct the airway and cause breathing difficulties.

When you are examining a casualty with a facial injury, assume that there is damage to the skull, brain, or neck; don't dismiss the symptoms as just the bruising around an eye that is commonly known as a "black eye."

WHAT TO DO

1 Help the casualty sit down and make sure the airway is open and clear.

2 Ask the casualty to spit out any blood, displaced teeth, or dentures from his mouth. Put any teeth in milk to send to the hospital with him.

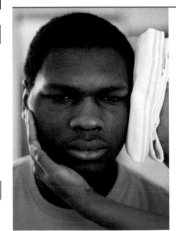

3 Gently place a cold compress (p.241) against the casualty's face to help reduce pain and minimize swelling. Treat for shock (pp.112–13) if necessary.

4 Call **911** for emergency help.

5 Monitor and record vital signs—level of response, breathing, and pulse (pp.52–53)—while waiting for help to arrive.

SEE ALSO Head injury **pp.144–45** | Knocked-out adult tooth **p.125** | Shock **pp.112–13** | Spinal injury **pp.157–59** | The unconscious casualty **pp.54–87**

LOWER JAW INJURY

Jaw fractures are usually the result of direct force, such as a heavy blow to the chin. In some situations, a blow to one side of the jaw produces indirect force, which causes a fracture on the other side of the face. A fall onto the point of the chin can fracture the jaw on both sides. The lower jaw may also be dislocated by a blow to the face, or is sometimes dislocated by yawning.

If the face is seriously injured, with the jaw fractured in more than one place, treat as for a facial injury (opposite).

RECOGNITION

There may be:

- Difficulty speaking, swallowing, and moving the jaw
- Pain and nausea when moving the jaw
- Displaced or loose teeth and dribbling from the mouth
- Swelling and bruising inside and outside the mouth

WHAT TO DO

1 If the casualty is not seriously injured, help him sit with his head forward to allow fluids to drain from his mouth. Encourage the casualty to spit out loose teeth, and keep them to send to the hospital with him.

2 Give the casualty a soft pad to hold firmly against his jaw in order to support it.

3 Arrange to take or send the casualty to the hospital. Keep his jaw supported throughout.

YOUR AIMS

- To protect the airway
- To arrange transportation to the hospital

CHEEKBONE AND NOSE INJURY

Fractures of the cheekbone and nose are usually the result of direct blows to the face. Swollen facial tissues are likely to cause discomfort, and the air passages in the nose may become blocked, making breathing difficult. These injuries should always be examined in the hospital.

CAUTION

- If there is clear fluid or watery blood leaking from the casualty's nose, treat the casualty as for a head injury (p.144–45).
- Do not allow the casualty to eat or drink because an anesthetic may be needed.

WHAT TO DO

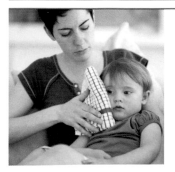

1 Gently place a cold compress, such as a cold pad or ice pack (p.241), against the injured area to help reduce pain and minimize swelling.

2 If the casualty has a nosebleed, try to pinch the nose to stop the bleeding (p.124). Arrange to take or send the casualty to the hospital.

RECOGNITION

There may be:

- Pain, swelling and bruising
- Obvious wound or bleeding from the nose or mouth

YOUR AIMS

- To minimize pain and swelling
- To arrange transportation to the hospital.

COLLARBONE INJURY

RECOGNITION

There may be:

- Pain and tenderness, increased by movement
- Swelling and deformity of the shoulder
- Attempts by the casualty to relax muscles and relieve pain; she may support her arm at the elbow, and incline her head to her injured side

YOUR AIMS

- To immobilize the injured shoulder and arm
- To arrange transportation to the hospital

The collarbones (clavicles) form "struts" between the shoulder blades and the top of the breastbone to help support the arms. It is rare for a collarbone to be broken by a direct blow. Usually, a fracture results from an indirect force transmitted from an impact at the shoulder or passing along the arm, for example, from a fall onto an outstretched arm. Collarbone fractures often occur in young people as a result of sports activities. The broken ends of the collarbone may be displaced, causing swelling and bleeding in the surrounding tissues as well as distortion of the shoulder.

WHAT TO DO

1 **Help the casualty** sit down. Gently place the injured arm across her body in the position that she finds most comfortable. Ask her to support the elbow on the injured side with her other hand, or help her do it.

2 **Support the arm** on the affected side with an arm sling (p.251). Make sure the knot is clear of the site of injury.

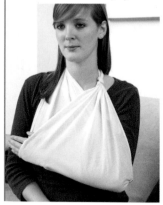

3 **For extra support,** secure the arm to the chest by tying a broad-fold bandage (p.249) around the chest and the sling. Once the arm is supported, the casualty will be more comfortable.

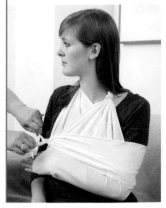

4 **Arrange to take or send** the casualty to the hospital in the position she finds most comfortable.

SHOULDER INJURY

A fall onto the shoulder or an outstretched arm or a wrenching force may pull the head of the upper arm bone (humerus) out of the joint socket—dislocation of the shoulder. At the same time, ligaments around the shoulder joint may be torn. This injury can be very painful. Some people experience repeated dislocations and may need a strengthening operation on the affected shoulder.

A fall onto the point of the shoulder may damage the ligaments that brace the collarbone at the shoulder. Other shoulder injuries include damage to the joint capsule and to the tendons around the shoulder; these injuries tend to be common in older people. To treat a shoulder sprain, rest the affected part, cool the injury with ice, and use a sling to provide comfortable support.

CAUTION

- Do not attempt to replace a dislocated bone into its socket.
- Do not allow the casualty to eat or drink because an anesthetic may be needed.

RECOGNITION

There may be:

- Severe pain, increased by movement; the pain may make the casualty reluctant to move
- Attempts by the casualty to relieve pain by supporting the arm and inclining the head to the injured side
- A flat, angular look to the shoulder

YOUR AIMS

- To support and immobilize the injured limb
- To arrange transportation to the hospital

WHAT TO DO

1 **Help the casualty** sit down. Gently place the arm on the injured side across her body in the position that is most comfortable. Ask the casualty to support her elbow on the injured side, or help her do it.

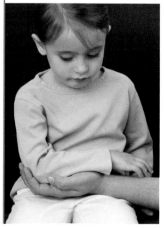

2 **Support the arm** on the injured side with an arm sling (p.251).

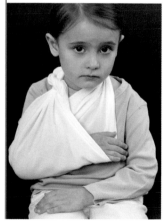

3 **For extra support** if necessary, secure the arm to the chest by tying a broad-fold bandage (p.249) around the chest and the sling.

4 **Arrange to take or send** the casualty to the hospital in the position she finds most comfortable.

SEE ALSO Fractures pp.136–38

UPPER ARM INJURY

RECOGNITION

There may be:

- Pain, increased by movement
- Tenderness and deformity over the site of a fracture
- Rapid swelling
- Bruising, which may develop more slowly

YOUR AIMS

- To immobilize the arm
- To arrange transportation to the hospital

A serious form of upper arm injury is a fracture of the long bone in the upper arm (humerus). The bone may be fractured across the center by a direct blow. However, it is much more common, especially in elderly people, for the arm bone to break at the shoulder end, usually in a fall.

A fracture at the top of the bone is usually a stable injury (p.136) because the broken bone ends stay in place. For this reason, it may not be immediately apparent that the bone is broken, although the arm is likely to be painful. There is a possibility that the casualty will cope with the pain and leave the fracture untreated for some time.

WHAT TO DO

1 **Help the casualty sit** down. Remove all jewelry such as bracelets, rings, and watches. Gently place the forearm horizontally across her body in the position that is most comfortable. Ask her to support her elbow if possible.

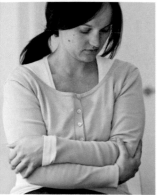

2 **Slide a triangular bandage** in position between the arm and the chest, ready to make an arm sling (p.251). Place soft padding between the injured arm and the body, then support the arm and its padding in an arm sling.

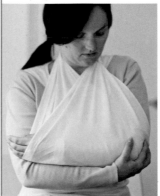

3 **For extra support,** or if the trip to the hospital is prolonged, secure the arm by tying a broad-fold bandage (p.249) around the chest and over the sling; make sure that the broad-fold bandage is below the fracture site.

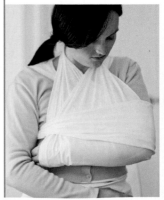

4 **Arrange to take or send the** casualty to the hospital.

ELBOW INJURY

Fractures or dislocations at the elbow usually result from a fall onto the hand. Children often fracture the upper arm bone just above the elbow. This is an unstable fracture (p.136), and the bone ends may damage blood vessels. Circulation in the arm needs to be checked regularly. In any elbow injury, the elbow will be stiff and difficult to straighten. Never try to force a casualty to bend it.

WHAT TO DO

1 If the elbow can be bent, treat as for upper arm injury opposite. Remove all jewelry such as bracelets, rings, and watches.

2 If the casualty cannot bend her arm, help her sit down. Place padding, such as a towel, around the elbow for comfort and support.

3 Secure the arm in the most comfortable position for the casualty using broad-fold bandages. Keep the bandages clear of the fracture site.

RECOGNITION

There may be:

■ Pain, increased by movement

■ Tenderness over the site of a fracture

■ Swelling, bruising, and deformity

■ Fixed elbow

YOUR AIMS

■ To immobilize the arm without further injury to the joint

■ To arrange transportation to the hospital

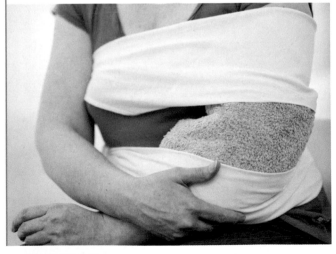

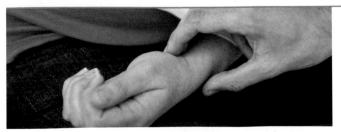

4 Arrange to take or send the casualty to the hospital.

5 Check the wrist pulse (p.53) in the injured arm every ten minutes until medical help arrives. If you cannot feel a pulse, gently undo the bandages and straighten the arm until the pulse returns. Support the arm in this position.

FOREARM AND WRIST INJURIES

RECOGNITION

There may be:

- Pain, increased by movement
- Swelling, bruising, and deformity
- Possible bleeding with an open fracture

YOUR AIMS

- To immobilize the arm
- To arrange transportation to the hospital

The bones of the forearm (radius and ulna) can be fractured by an impact such as a heavy blow or a fall. Because the bones have little fleshy covering, the broken ends may pierce the skin, producing an open fracture (p.136).

A fall onto an outstretched hand can result in various types of fractures of the wrist. One type, Colles fractures, commonly occurs in elderly people.

The wrist joint is rarely dislocated but is often sprained. It can be difficult to distinguish between a sprain and a fracture, especially if the tiny scaphoid bone (at the base of the thumb) is injured. If you are in any doubt about the injury treat as a fracture.

WHAT TO DO

1 **Ask the casualty to sit down.** Steady and support the injured forearm and place it across his body; ask the casualty to support it if he can. Expose and treat any wound, and remove jewelry, especially watches, bracelets, and rings.

2 **Slide a triangular bandage** in position between the arm and the chest, ready to make an arm sling (p.251). Surround the forearm in soft padding, such as a small towel.

3 **Support the arm** and the padding with an arm sling; make sure the knot is tied on the injured side.

4 **For extra support,** or if the trip to the hospital is likely to be prolonged, secure the arm to the body by tying a swathe (p.251) over the sling and body. Position the bandage as close to the elbow as you can. Arrange to take or send the casualty to the hospital.

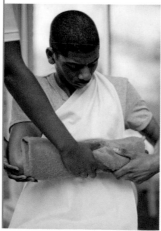

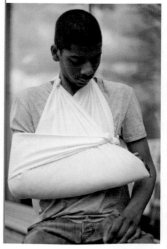

| SEE ALSO Fractures **pp.136–38** | Severe external bleeding **pp.114–15**

HAND AND FINGER INJURIES

The bones and joints in the hand can suffer various types of injury, such as fractures, cuts, and bruising. Minor fractures are usually caused by direct force. A fracture of the knuckle often results from a punch.

Multiple fractures, affecting many or all of the bones in the hand, are usually caused by crushing injuries. The fractures may be open, with bleeding and swelling, needing immediate first aid treatment.

The joints in the fingers or thumb are sometimes dislocated or sprained as a result of a fall onto the hand (for example, while someone is skiing or ice skating).

Always compare the suspected fractured hand with the uninjured hand because finger fractures result in deformities that may not be immediately obvious.

CAUTION

- Do not allow the casualty to eat or drink because an anesthetic may be needed.

RECOGNITION

There may be:
- Pain, increased by movement
- Swelling, bruising, and deformity
- Possible bleeding with an open fracture

YOUR AIMS

- To elevate the hand and immobilize it
- To arrange transportation to the hospital

WHAT TO DO

1 **Help the casualty** sit down and ask her to raise and support the affected wrist and hand; help her if necessary. Treat any bleeding and losely cover the wound with a sterile dressing or large clean, gauze pad.

2 **Remove any rings,** bracelets, and watch before the hand begins to swell, and keep it raised to minimize swelling. Wrap the hand in soft, nonfluffy padding for extra protection.

3 **Gently support** the affected arm across the casualty's body by placing it in an elevation sling (p.252).

4 **For extra support,** or if the trip to the hospital is likely to be prolonged, secure the arm by tying a broad-fold bandage (p.249) around the chest and over the sling; keep it away from the injury. Arrange to take or send the casualty to the hospital.

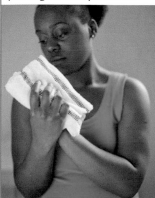

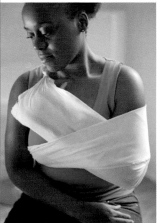

SEE ALSO Crush injury **p.118** | Dislocated joint **p.139** | Fractures **pp.136–38** | Wound to the palm **p.127**

RIB INJURY

CAUTION

- Do not allow the casualty to eat or drink because an anesthetic may be needed.
- If the casualty loses consciousness, position him on the ground, on his back with his airway open. If he is not breathing, begin CPR with chest compressions (pp.54–87). If he needs to be placed in the recovery position, lay him on his injured side to allow the lung on the uninjured side to work to its full capacity.

One or more ribs can be fractured by direct force to the chest from a blow or a fall, or by a crush injury (p.118). If there is a wound over the fracture, or if a broken rib pierces a lung, the casualty's breathing may be seriously impaired.

An injury to the chest can cause an area of fractured ribs to become detached from the rest of the chest wall, producing what is called a "flail-chest" injury. The detached area moves inward when the casualty inhales, and outward as he exhales. This so-called "paradoxical" breathing causes severe breathing difficulties.

Fractures of the lower ribs may injure internal organs such as the liver and spleen, and may cause internal bleeding.

RECOGNITION

- Bruising, swelling, or a wound at the fracture site
- Pain at the site of injury
- Pain on taking a deep breath
- Shallow breathing
- A wound over the fracture; you may hear air being "sucked" into chest cavity
- Paradoxical breathing
- Signs of internal bleeding (p.116) and shock (pp.112–13)

YOUR AIMS

- To support the chest wall
- To arrange transportation to the hospital

WHAT TO DO

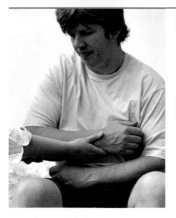

1 Help the casualty sit down and ask him to support the arm on the injured side; help him if necessary. For extra support place the arm on the injured side in a sling (pp.251–52).

2 Arrange to take or send the casualty to the hospital.

SPECIAL CASE A PENETRATING CHEST WOUND

If there is a penetrating wound, help the casualty sit down on the floor, leaning toward the injured side. Cover and seal the wound on three edges (pp.104–05). Support him with cushions and place the arm on the injured side in an elevation sling (p.252). **Call 911 for emergency help.** Monitor and record vital signs—level of response, breathing, and pulse (pp.52–53)—while waiting for help to arrive.

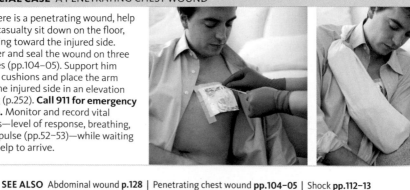

FRACTURED PELVIS

Injuries to the pelvis are usually caused by indirect force, such as a car crash, a fall from a height, or by crushing. These incidents can force the head of the thigh bone (femur) through the hip socket in the pelvis.

A fracture of the pelvic bones may also be complicated by injury to tissues and organs inside the pelvis, such as the bladder and the urinary passages. The bleeding from large organs and blood vessels in the pelvis may be severe and lead to shock.

WHAT TO DO

1 Help the casualty lie down on her back with her head flat or low to minimize shock. Keep her legs straight and flat or, if it is more comfortable, help her bend her knees slightly and support them with padding, such as a cushion or folded clothing.

2 Place padding between the bony points of her knees and ankles. Immobilize her legs by bandaging them together with folded triangular bandages (p.249); secure her feet and ankles with a narrow-fold bandage (1), and the knees with a broad-fold bandage (2).

3 Call 911 for emergency help. Treat the casualty for shock (pp.112–13). Do not raise the legs.

4 Monitor and record vital signs—level of response, breathing, and pulse (pp.52–53) —until help arrives.

CAUTION

- Do not allow the casualty to eat or drink because an anesthetic may be needed.
- Keep movements of the casualty to a minimum to prevent worsening the injury.
- Do not bandage the casualty's legs together if this increases the pain. In such cases, only surround the injured area with soft padding, such as clothing or towels.

RECOGNITION

There may be:

- An inability to walk or even stand, although the legs appear uninjured
- Pain and tenderness in the region of the hip, groin, or back, which increases with movement
- Difficulty or pain when urinating, and bloodstained clothing
- Signs of shock and internal bleeding

YOUR AIMS

- To minimize the risk of shock
- To arrange urgent removal to the hospital

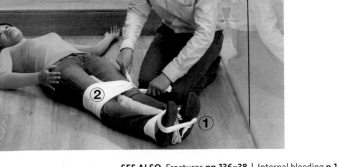

BACK PAIN

Lower back pain is common and most adults may experience it at some point in their lives. It may be acute (sudden onset) or chronic (long term). It is usually caused by age-related degenerative changes or results from minor injury affecting muscles, ligaments, vertebrae, disks, or nerves. It may be the result of heavy manual work, a fall, or a turning or twisting movement. Serious conditions causing back pain are rare and beyond the scope of first aid.

Most cases are simple muscular backaches, often in the lower back. In some casualties, the pain may extend down one leg. This is called sciatica and is caused by pressure on the nerve root (a so-called "pinched nerve").

Back pain that results from more serious mechanisms of injury may indicate spinal injury and requires investigation and treatment (see Spinal injury, pp.157–59).

RECOGNITION

- Pain in the lower back following lifting or manual work
- Possible pain radiating down the back of one leg with numbness or tingling in the affected leg—sciatica

YOUR AIM

- To relieve pain

WHAT TO DO

1 **For minor back pain, advise the casualty** to stay active to mobilize the injured area. Encourage him to return to normal activity as soon as possible.

2 **An adult casualty may** take the recommended dose of acetaminophen or ibuprofen tablets, or his own pain medicine.

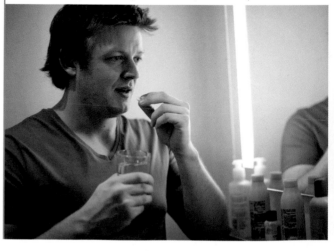

3 **For disabling back pain with neurological symptoms** (pp.157–59), arrange transportation to a hospital.

SPINAL INJURY

Injuries to the spine can involve one or more parts of the back and/or neck: the bones (vertebrae), the disks of tissue that separate the vertebrae, the surrounding muscles, and ligaments, or the spinal cord and the nerves that branch off from it.

The most serious risk associated with spinal injury is damage to the spinal cord. Such damage can cause loss of power and/or sensation below the injured area. The spinal cord or nerve roots can suffer temporary damage if they are pinched by displaced or dislocated disks, or by fragments of broken bone. If the cord is partly or completely severed, damage may be permanent.

The most important indicator is the mechanism of the injury. Suspect spinal injury if abnormal forces have been exerted on the back or neck, and particularly if a casualty complains of any changes in sensation or difficulties with movement. If the incident involved violent forward or backward bending, or twisting of the spine, you must assume that the casualty has a spinal injury. You must take particular care to avoid unnecessary movement of the head, neck, and spine at all times.

Although spinal cord injury may occur without any damage to the vertebrae, spinal fracture greatly increases the risk. The areas that are most vulnerable are the bones in the neck and those in the lower back.

Any of the following incidents should alert you to a possible spinal injury:

- **Falling from a height,** such as a ladder
- **Falling awkwardly,** for instance, while doing gymnastics or bouncing on a trampoline
- **Diving into a shallow pool** and hitting the bottom
- **Falling from a horse** or motorcycle
- **Football tackle or misplaced** hit
- **Sudden deceleration** in a motor vehicle
- **A heavy object falling** across the back
- **Injury to the head** or the face

Spinal cord protection
The spinal cord is protected by the bony vertebral (spinal) column. Nerves branching from the cord emerge between adjacent vertebrae.

RECOGNITION

When the vertebrae are damaged, there may be:

- Pain in the neck or back at the injury site. This may be masked by other, more painful, injuries.
- Irregularity or twisting in the normal curve of the spine
- Tenderness and/or bruising in the skin over the spine

When the spinal cord is damaged, there may be:

- Loss of control over limbs movement may be weak or absent
- Loss of sensation, or abnormal sensations such as burning or tingling; a casualty may tell you that his limbs feel stiff, heavy, or clumsy
- Loss of bladder and/or bowel control
- Breathing difficulties

Spinal cord

Nerve root

Vertebra

Intervertebral disk

◀◀ SPINAL INJURY

YOUR AIMS

- To prevent further injury
- To arrange urgent removal to the hospital

WHAT TO DO FOR A CONSCIOUS CASUALTY

 1 Reassure the casualty and advise him not to move. **Call 911 for emergency help,** or ask a helper to do this.

2 Kneel or lie behind the casualty's head. Rest your elbows on the ground or on your knees to keep your arms steady. Grasp the sides of the casualty's head. Spread your fingers so that you do not cover his ears, so he can hear you. Steady and support his head in this neutral position, in which the head, neck, and spine are aligned.

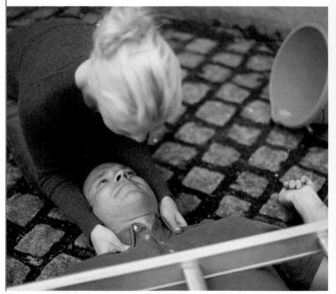

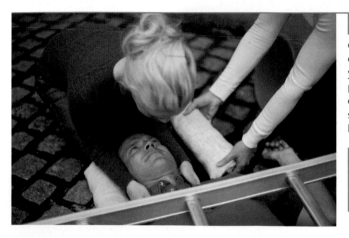

3 Ask a helper to place rolled-up blankets, towels, or items of clothing on either side of the casualty's head and neck, while you keep his head in the neutral position. Continue to support the casualty's head until emergency services take over, no matter how long this may be.

4 Get your helper to monitor and record vital signs—level of response, breathing, and pulse (pp.52–53)—while waiting for help to arrive.

WHAT TO DO FOR AN UNCONSCIOUS CASUALTY

1 **Kneel or lie behind the casualty's head.** Rest your elbows on the ground or on your knees to keep your arms steady. Grasp the sides of her head. Support her head so that her head, trunk, and legs are in a straight line.

2 **Open the casualty's airway** using the jaw-thrust technique. Place your fingertips at the angles of her jaw. Gently lift the jaw to open the airway. Take care not to tilt the casualty's neck.

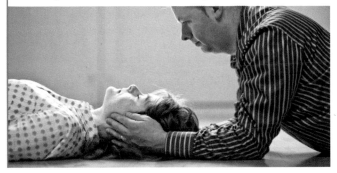

YOUR AIMS

- To maintain an open airway
- To begin CPR if necessary
- To prevent further spinal damage
- To arrange urgent removal to the hospital

3 **Check the casualty's breathing.** If she is breathing, continue to support her head. **Call 911 for emergency help** or ask a helper to do this.

4 **If the casualty is not breathing,** begin CPR (pp.66–67). If you need to turn the casualty, use the log-roll technique (below).

5 **Monitor and record vital signs**—level of response, breathing, and pulse (pp.52–53)—while waiting for help.

SPECIAL CASE LOG-ROLL TECHNIQUE

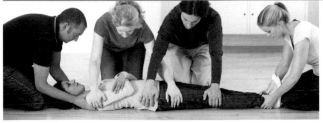

1 **This technique** should be used to turn a casualty who has a suspected spinal injury. Position the casualty and rescuers as shown, with the casualty's arms crossed over chest. The person securing the head will give the command to roll once everyone is in proper position.

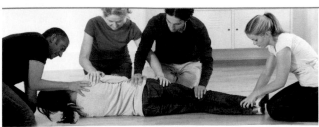

2 **Direct your helpers** to roll the casualty in the agreed-upon direction (in case she vomits, for example). Keep the casualty's head, trunk, and legs in a straight line at all times; the upper leg should be supported in a slightly raised position to keep the spine straight.

HIP AND THIGH INJURIES

RECOGNITION

There may be:

- Pain at the site of the injury
- An inability to walk
- Signs of shock
- Shortening of the leg and turning outward of the knee and foot

YOUR AIMS

- To immobilize the limb
- To arrange urgent removal to the hospital

The most serious injury of the thighbone (femur) is a fracture. It takes a considerable force, such as a car crash or a fall from a height, to fracture the shaft of the femur. This is a serious injury because the broken bone ends can pierce major blood vessels, causing severe blood loss, and shock may result.

Fracture of the neck of the femur is common in elderly people, particularly women, whose bones become less dense and more brittle with age (osteoporosis). This fracture is usually a stable injury in which the bone ends are impacted together. The casualty may be able to walk with a fractured neck of the femur for some time before the fracture is discovered. In the hip joint, the most serious, although much less common, type of injury is dislocation.

SPECIAL CASE PREPARING FOR TRANSPORTATION

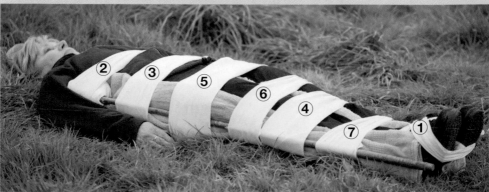

If the trip to the hospital is likely to be long and rough, more sturdy support for the leg and feet will be needed. Use a specially made malleable splint or a long, solid object, such as a fence post or long walking stick, which reaches from the armpit to the foot. Place the splint against the injured side. Insert padding between the casualty's legs and between the splint and her body. Tie the feet together with a narrow-fold bandage (1). Secure the splint to the body with broad-fold bandages in the following order: at the chest (2), pelvis (3), knees (4), above and below the fracture site (5 and 6), and at one extra point (7). Do not bandage over the fracture site. Once the casualty's leg is fully immobilized, she should be moved onto the stretcher using the log-roll technique (p.159).

WHAT TO DO

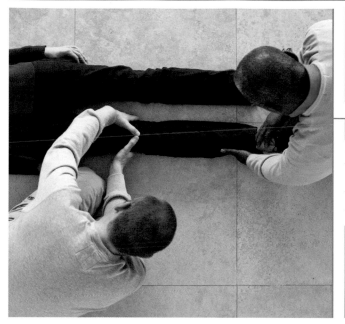

1 **Help the casualty** lie down. Ask a helper to gently steady and support the injured limb at the knee. For a hip dislocation, place a pillow under the knee if this makes the casualty more comfortable.

2 **Call 911 for emergency help.** If the ambulance is expected to arrive quickly, keep the leg supported in the same position (rather than trying to straighten it) until the ambulance arrives.

3 **For a femur fracture,** gently straighten the casualty's leg. If necessary, realign the limb (p.137). Support the limb at the ankle while you straighten it; pull gently in the line of the limb until the ambulance arrives.

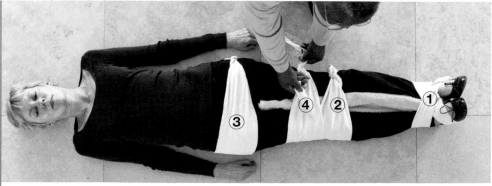

4 **If the ambulance** is not expected to arrive quickly, immobilize a femur fracture by securing it to the uninjured leg. Gently bring the uninjured leg alongside the injured one. Position a narrow-fold bandage (p.249) at the ankles and feet (1), then a broad-fold one at the knees (2). Add additional bandages above (3) and below (4) the fracture site. Place soft padding between the legs to prevent the bony parts from rubbing. Secure the bandages on the uninjured side.

5 **Take any steps possible** to treat the casualty for shock (pp.112–13): insulate her from the cold with blankets or clothing. Do not raise her legs.

LOWER LEG INJURIES

RECOGNITION

There may be:
- Localized pain
- Swelling, bruising, and deformity of the leg
- An open wound
- Inability to stand on the injured leg

YOUR AIMS

- To immobilize the leg
- To arrange transportation to the hospital

Injuries to the lower leg include fractures of the shinbone (tibia) and the fibula, as well as damage to the soft tissues (muscles, ligaments, and tendons).

Fractures of the tibia are usually due to a heavy blow (for example, from the bumper of a moving vehicle). Because there is little flesh over the tibia, a fracture is more likely to produce a wound. The fibula can be broken by the twisting forces that sprain an ankle.

WHAT TO DO

1 **Help the casualty lie down,** and gently steady and support the injured leg. If there is a wound, carefully expose it and treat the bleeding. Place a dressing over the wound to protect it.

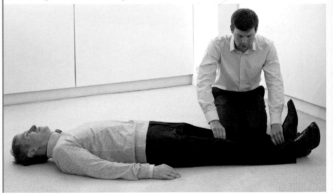

2 **Call 911 for emergency help.** Support the injured leg with your hands; hold the joints above and below the fracture site to prevent any movement. Maintain support until the ambulance arrives.

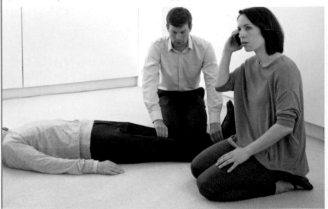

3 If the ambulance is delayed, support the injured leg by splinting it to the other leg. Bring the uninjured leg alongside the injured one and slide bandages under both legs. Position a narrow-fold bandage (p.249) at the feet and ankles (1), then broad-fold bandages at the knees (2) and above and below the fracture site (3 and 4). Insert padding between the lower legs. Tie a figure-eight bandage around the feet and ankles, then secure the other bandages, knotting them on the uninjured side.

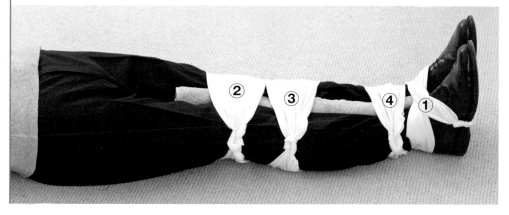

4 If the casualty's trip to the hospital is likely to be long and rough, place soft padding on the outside of the injured leg, from the knee to the foot. Secure the legs with broad-fold bandages as described above.

SPECIAL CASE IF THE FRACTURE IS NEAR THE ANKLE

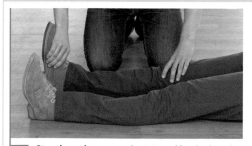

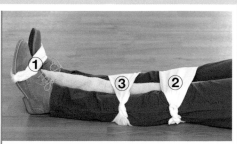

1 Steady and support the injured leg by hand at the knee and foot (not over the fracture site) to prevent any movement. If there is a wound, treat the bleeding and place a dressing over the wound to protect it. **Call 911 for emergency help.** Maintain support until the ambulance arrives.

2 If the ambulance is delayed, splint the injured leg to the other leg—ask a helper to maintain support while you secure bandages. Bring the uninjured leg to the injured one. Position a narrow-fold bandage (p.249) at the feet. Slide two broad-fold bandages under both knees; leave one at the knee (2) and slide the other down to just above the fracture site (3). Insert padding between the lower legs and tie the feet together (1). Then secure the other two bandages (2 then 3). Tie all knots on the uninjured side.

KNEE INJURY

RECOGNITION

There may be:
- Pain on attempting to move the knee
- Swelling at the knee joint

YOUR AIMS

- To protect the knee in the most comfortable position
- To arrange urgent removal to the hospital

The knee is the hinge joint between the thighbone (femur) and shinbone (tibia). It is capable of bending, straightening, and, in the bent position, slight rotation.

The knee joint is supported by strong muscles and ligaments and is protected at the front by a disk of bone called the kneecap (patella). Disks of cartilage protect the end surfaces of the major bones. Direct blows, violent twists, or sprains can damage these structures. Possible knee injuries include fracture or dislocation of the patella, sprains, and damage to the cartilage.

A knee injury may make it impossible for the casualty to bend the joint, and you should ensure that the casualty does not try to walk on the injured leg. Bleeding or fluid in the knee joint may cause marked swelling around the knee.

WHAT TO DO

1 Help the casualty lie down, preferably on a blanket to insulate him from the floor or ground. Place soft padding, such as pillows, blankets, or coats, under his injured knee to support it in the most comfortable position.

2 Apply an ice pack, then wrap soft padding around the joint. Secure padding with a roller bandage that extends from the middle of the lower leg to mid-thigh.

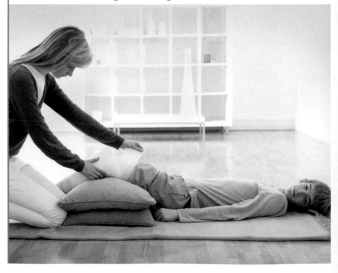

3 Call 911 for emergency help. The casualty needs to remain in the treatment position, so he should be transported to the hospital by ambulance.

ANKLE INJURY

A sprain is the most common ankle injury. It is usuallly caused by a twist to the ankle and can be treated using the **RICE** procedure (pp.140 41):

- Rest the affected part
- Cool the injury with Ice
- Provide comfortable Compression support with elastic bandaging
- Elevate the injury

If the casualty cannot bear any weight on the injured leg or there is severe pain, swelling, and/or deformity at the ankle, suspect a break and treat it as a fracture of the lower leg near the ankle (p.163). Be aware too, however, that a casualty may have a fracture and still be able to walk and move his toes. If you are in any doubt about an ankle injury, treat it as a fracture.

RECOGNITION

- Pain, increased either by movement or by putting weight on the foot
- Swelling at the site of injury

YOUR AIMS

- To relieve pain and swelling
- To obtain medical aid if necessary

WHAT TO DO

1 Support the ankle in the most comfortable position for the casualty, preferably raised.

2 Apply a cold compress, such as an ice pack or a cold pad (p.241), to the site to reduce swelling and bruising.

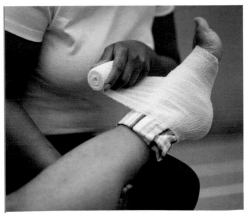

3 Apply comfortable support to the ankle. Leave the cold compress in place or wrap a layer of soft padding around the area. Bandage the ankle with a support bandage that extends from the base of the foot to the upper extent of the pain.

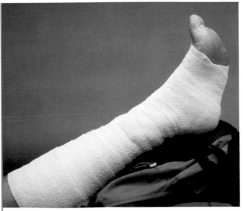

4 Raise and support the injured limb. Check the circulation beyond the bandaging (p.243) every ten minutes. If the circulation is impaired, loosen the bandage. If you suspect a broken bone, arrange to send the casualty to the hospital.

FOOT AND TOE INJURIES

RECOGNITION

- Difficulty in walking
- Stiffness of movement
- Bruising and swelling
- Deformity

YOUR AIMS

- To minimize swelling
- To arrange transportation to the hospital

The bones and joints in the foot can suffer various types of injury, such as fractures and dislocations, cuts, and bruising. Minor fractures are usually caused by direct force. Always compare the injured foot with the uninjured foot, especially toes, because fractures can result in deformities that may not be immediately obvious. Multiple fractures, affecting many or all of the bones in the foot, are usually caused by crushing injuries. These fractures may be open, with severe bleeding and swelling, needing immediate first aid treatment. Serious foot and toe injures must be treated in the hospital.

WHAT TO DO

1 Help the casualty lie down, and carefully steady and support the injured leg. If there is a wound, carefully expose it and treat the bleeding. Place a dressing over the wound to protect it.

2 Remove any foot jewelry before the area begins to swell.

3 Apply a cold compress, such as an ice pack or a cold pad (p.241). This will also help relieve swelling and reduce pain.

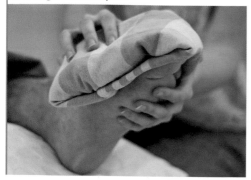

4 Place padding around the casualty's foot and bandage the ice pack firmly in place.

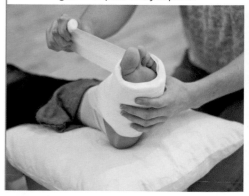

5 Arrange to take or send the casualty to the hospital. If he is not being transported by ambulance, try to ensure that the injured foot remains elevated during travel.

CRAMPS

This condition is a sudden painful spasm in one or more muscles. Cramps commonly occur during sleep. They can also develop after strenuous exercise, due to a buildup of chemical waste products in the muscles, or to excessive loss of salts and fluids from the body through sweating or dehydration. Cramps can often be relieved by stretching and massaging the affected muscles.

YOUR AIM

- To relieve the spasm and pain

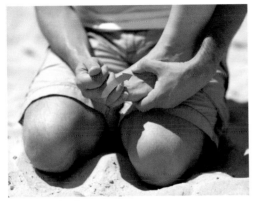

Cramp in the foot
Help the casualty stand with his weight on the front of his foot; you can also rest the foot on your knee to stretch the affected muscles. Once the spasm has passed, massage the affected part of the foot with your fingers.

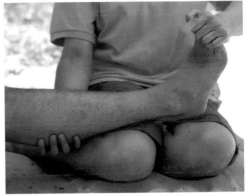

Cramp in the calf muscles
Help the casualty straighten his knee, and support his foot. Flex his foot upward toward his shin to stretch the calf muscles, then massage the affected area on the back of the calf.

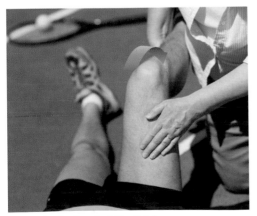

Cramp in the front of the thigh
Help the casualty lie down. Raise the leg and bend the knee to stretch the muscles. Massage the affected muscles once the spasm has passed.

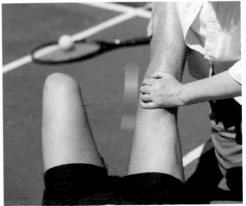

Cramp in the back of the thigh
Help the casualty lie down. Raise the leg and straighten the knee to stretch the muscles. Massage the area once the spasm has passed.

SEE ALSO Dehydration p.182 | Heat exhaustion p.184 |

8

This chapter deals with the effects of injuries and illnesses caused by environmental factors such as extremes of heat and cold.

The skin protects the body and helps maintain body temperature within a normal range. It can be damaged by fire, hot liquids, or caustic substances. This chapter contains advice on how to assess burns, whether minor or severe.

The effects of temperature extremes can also impair skin and other body functions. Injuries may be localized—such as frostbite or sunburn—or generalized, as in heat exhaustion or hypothermia. Young children and the elderly are most susceptible to problems caused by extremes of temperature.

AIMS AND OBJECTIVES

- To assess the casualty's condition quickly and calmly.
- To comfort and reassure the casualty.
- To call 911 for emergency help if you suspect a serious illness or injury.
- To be aware of your own needs.

For burns:
- To protect yourself and the casualty from danger;
- To assess the burn, prevent further damage, and relieve symptoms.

For extremes of temperature:
- To protect the casualty from heat or cold.
- To restore normal body temperature.

EFFECTS OF
HEAT AND COLD

THE SKIN

One of the largest organs, the skin plays key roles in protecting the body from injury and infection and in maintaining the body at a constant temperature.

The skin consists of two layers of tissue—an outer layer (epidermis) and an inner layer (dermis)—that lie on a layer of fatty tissue (subcutaneous fat). The top part of the epidermis is made up of dead, flattened skin cells, which are constantly shed and replaced by new cells made in the lower part of this layer. The epidermis is protected by an oily substance called sebum—secreted from glands called sebaceous glands—which keeps the skin supple and waterproof.

The lower layer of the skin, the dermis, contains the blood vessels, nerves, muscles, sebaceous glands, sweat glands, and hair roots (follicles). The ends of sensory nerves within the dermis register sensations from the body's surface, such as heat, cold, pain, and even the slightest touch. Blood vessels supply the skin with nutrients and help regulate body temperature by preserving or releasing heat (opposite).

Structure of the skin

The skin is made up of two layers: the thin, outer epidermis and the thicker dermis beneath it. Most of the structures of the skin, such as blood vessels, nerves, and hair roots, are contained within the dermis.

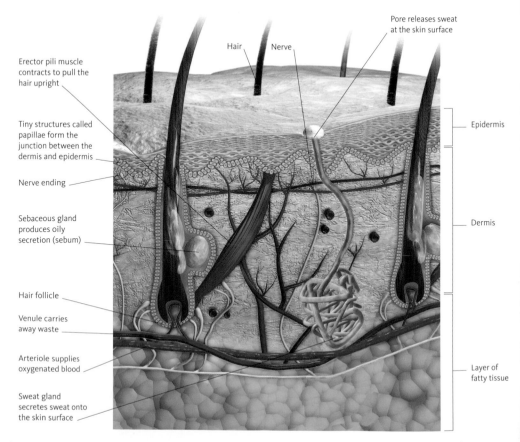

Erector pili muscle contracts to pull the hair upright

Tiny structures called papillae form the junction between the dermis and epidermis

Nerve ending

Sebaceous gland produces oily secretion (sebum)

Hair follicle

Venule carries away waste

Arteriole supplies oxygenated blood

Sweat gland secretes sweat onto the skin surface

Hair

Nerve

Pore releases sweat at the skin surface

Epidermis

Dermis

Layer of fatty tissue

MAINTAINING BODY TEMPERATURE

One of the major functions of the skin is to help maintain the body temperature within its optimum range of 97–99°F (36–37°C). A structure in the brain called the hypothalamus regulates body temperature. If the temperature of blood passing through this thermostat falls or rises to a level outside the optimum range, various mechanisms are activated to either warm or cool the body as necessary.

HOW THE BODY KEEPS WARM

When the body becomes too cold, changes take place to prevent heat from escaping. Blood vessels at the body surface narrow (constrict) to keep warm blood in the main part (core) of the body. The activity of the sweat glands is reduced, and hairs stand on end to "trap" warm air close to the skin. In addition to the

mechanisms that prevent heat loss, other body systems act to produce more warmth. The rate of metabolism is increased. Heat is also generated by muscle activity, which may be either voluntary (for example, during physical exercise) or, in cold conditions, involuntary (shivering).

HOW THE BODY LOSES HEAT

In hot conditions, the body activates a number of mechanisms to encourage heat loss and thus prevent the body temperature from becoming too high. Blood vessels that lie in or just under the skin widen (dilate). As a result, blood flow to the body surface increases and more heat is lost. In addition, the sweat glands become more active and secrete more sweat. This sweat then cools the skin as it evaporates.

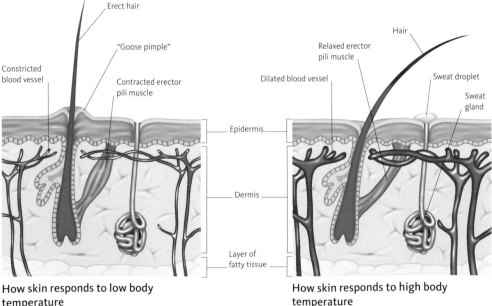

Erect hair

"Goose pimple"

Constricted blood vessel

Contracted erector pili muscle

Relaxed erector pili muscle

Dilated blood vessel

Hair

Sweat droplet

Sweat gland

Epidermis

Dermis

Layer of fatty tissue

How skin responds to low body temperature
Blood vessels narrow (constrict) to reduce blood flow to the skin. The erector pili muscles contract, making the hairs stand upright and trap warm air close to the skin.

How skin responds to high body temperature
Blood vessels widen (dilate), making the skin appear flushed, and heat is lost. Sweat glands become active and produce sweat droplets, which evaporate and cool the skin.

ASSESSING A BURN

When skin is damaged by burning, it can no longer function effectively as a natural barrier against infection. In addition, body fluid may be lost because tiny blood vessels in the skin leak tissue fluid (serum). This fluid either collects under the skin to form blisters or leaks through the surface.

There may be related injuries, significant fluid loss, and infection may develop later.

WHAT TO ASSESS

It is particularly important to consider the circumstances in which the burn has occurred; whether or not the airway is likely to have been affected; and the extent, location, and depth of the burn.

There are many possible causes of burns (below). By establishing the cause of the burn, you may be able to identify any other potential problems that could result. For example, a fire in an enclosed space is likely to have produced poisonous carbon monoxide gas, or other toxic fumes may have been released if burning material was involved. If the casualty's airway has been affected, he may have difficulty breathing and will need urgent medical attention and admission to the hospital.

The extent of the burn will also indicate whether or not shock is likely to develop. Shock is a life-threatening condition and occurs whenever there is a serious loss of body fluids (p.116). In a burn that covers a large area of the body, fluid loss will be significant and the risk of shock high.

If the burn is on a limb, fluid may collect in the tissues around it, causing swelling and pain. This buildup of fluid is particularly serious if the limb is constricted, for example by clothing or footwear.

Burns allow germs to enter the skin and therefore carry a serious risk of infection.

TYPES OF BURN AND POSSIBLE CAUSES

TYPE OF BURN	CAUSES
Dry burn	■ Flames ■ Contact with hot objects, such as domestic appliances or cigarettes
Scald	■ Steam ■ Hot liquids, such as tea and coffee, or hot oil
Electrical burn	■ Low-voltage current, as used by domestic appliances ■ High-voltage currents, as carried in overhead or underground cables ■ Lightning strikes
Radiation burn	■ Sunburn ■ Overexposure to ultraviolet rays from a sunlamp ■ Exposure to a radioactive source, such as an X-ray
Chemical burn	■ Industrial chemicals, including inhaled fumes and corrosive gases ■ Domestic chemicals and agents, such as paint stripper, caustic soda, weed killers, bleach, oven cleaner, or any other strong acid or alkali chemical
Cold injury	■ Frostbite ■ Contact with freezing metals ■ Contact with freezing vapors, such as liquid oxygen or liquid nitrogen

DEPTH OF BURNS

Burns are classified according to the depth of skin damage. There are three depths: superficial, partial-thickness, and full-thickness. A casualty may suffer one or more depths of burn in a single incident.

A superficial burn involves only the outermost layer of skin, the epidermis. It usually heals well if first aid is given promptly and if blisters do not form. Sunburn is one of the most common types of superficial burn. Other causes include minor domestic incidents. Partial-thickness burns are very painful. They destroy the epidermis and cause the skin to become red and blistered. They usually heal well, but if they affect more than 20 percent of the body in an adult and 10 percent in a child, they can be life-threatening.

In full-thickness burns, pain sensation is lost, which masks the severity of the injury. The skin may look waxy, pale, or charred and needs urgent medical attention. There are likely to be areas of partial and superficial burns around them.

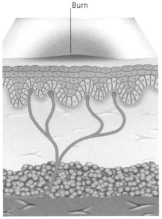

Burn

Superficial burn
This type of burn involves only the outermost layer of skin. Superficial burns are characterized by redness, swelling, and tenderness.

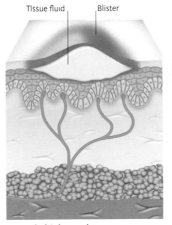

Tissue fluid   Blister

Partial-thickness burn
This affects the epidermis, and the skin becomes red and raw. Blisters form over the skin due to fluid released from the damaged tissues beneath.

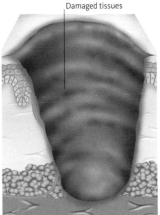

Damaged tissues

Full-thickness burn
With this type of burn, all the layers of the skin are affected; there may be some damage to nerves, fat tissue, muscles, and blood vessels.

BURNS THAT REQUIRE HOSPITAL TREATMENT

If the casualty is a child, seek medical advice or take the child to the hospital, however small the burn appears. For adults, medical attention should be sought for any serious burn. Such burns include:

- **All partial-thickness burns larger than** 10 **percent** of the total body surface area
- **All burns involving the face, hands, feet,** genitals and genital area, or major joints
- **All full-thickness burns**
- **Electrical burns,** including lightning injury
- **Chemical burns**
- **Inhalation injury**
- **Casualties with preexisting medical disorders** that could complicate treatment
- **Casualties with trauma as well as burns**
- **Casualties who will require** social, emotional, or rehabilitative treatment

If you are unsure about the severity of any burn, seek medical advice.

SEVERE BURNS AND SCALDS

CAUTION

- Do not remove anything sticking to the burn; you may cause further damage and introduce infection into the burned area.
- Do not burst any blisters.
- Do not apply any lotion or ointment to the burned area; it may damage tissues and increase the risk of infection.
- The use of specialized dressings, sprays, and gels to cool burns is not recommended.
- Do not use adhesive dressings or apply adhesive tape to the skin; a burn may be more extensive than it first appears.
- If the casualty has a burn on his face, do not cover the injury—you could cause the casualty distress and obstruct the airway.
- Do not allow the casualty to eat or drink because he may need an anesthetic.

RECOGNITION

There may be:

- Possible areas of superficial, partial thickness, and/or full-thickness burns
- Pain
- Difficulty breathing
- Signs of shock (pp.112–13)

YOUR AIMS

- To stop the burning and relieve pain
- To maintain an open airway
- To treat associated injuries
- To minimize the risk of infection
- To minimize the risk of shock
- To arrange urgent removal to the hospital
- To gather information for the emergency services

Take great care when treating thermal burns that are deep or extensive. The longer the burning continues, the more severe the injury will be. If the casualty has been injured in a fire, assume that smoke or hot air has also affected his airway and/or lungs.

Your priorities are to cool the burn (which stops the burning process and relieves the pain) and to monitor his breathing. A casualty with a severe burn or scald injury will almost certainly be suffering from shock because of the fluid loss and will need urgent hospital treatment.

The possibility of nonaccidental injury must always be considered, no matter what the age of the casualty. Keep an accurate record of what has happened and any treatment you have given. If you have to remove or cut away clothing, keep it in case of future investigation.

WHAT TO DO

1 Start cooling the burn as soon as possible after the injury occurred. Flood the burn with plenty of cool tap water, but do not delay removal of the casualty to the hospital. Help the casualty sit or lie down. If possible, try to prevent the burned area from coming into contact with the ground.

2 Call 911 for emergency help; if possible, get someone to do this while you cool the burn.

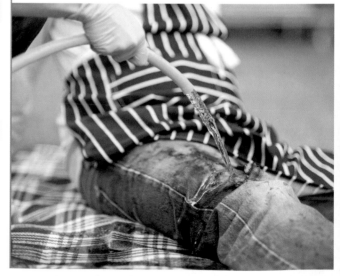

3 Continue cooling the affected area for at least ten minutes, or until the pain is relieved. Watch for signs of breathing difficulty. Do not overcool the casualty because you may lower the body temperature to a dangerous level. This is a particular hazard for babies and elderly people.

4 Do not touch or otherwise interfere with the burn. Gently remove rings, watches, belts, shoes, and burned or or smoldering clothing before the tissues begin to swell. A helper can do this while you are cooling the burn. Do not remove clothing that is stuck to the burn.

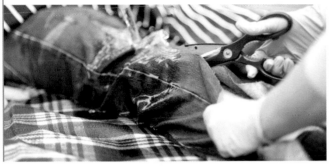

5 When the burn is cooled, cover the injured area with plastic wrap to protect it from infection. Discard the first two turns from the roll and then wrap it lengthwise over the burn. A clean plastic bag can be used to cover a hand or foot; secure it with a bandage or adhesive tape applied over the plastic, not the damaged skin. If there is no plastic wrap available, use a sterile nonstick dressing, or improvise with gauze. Apply any dressing very loosely.

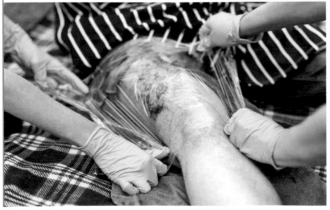

6 Reassure the casualty and treat him for shock (pp.112–13) if necessary. Record details of the casualty's injuries. Monitor and record his vital signs—level of response, breathing, and pulse (pp.52–53)—while waiting for emergency help to arrive.

MINOR BURNS AND SCALDS

RECOGNITION

- Reddened skin
- Pain in the area of the burn

Later there may be:

- Blistering of the affected skin

YOUR AIMS

- To stop the burning
- To relieve pain and swelling
- To minimize the risk of infection

SPECIAL CASE BLISTERS

Never burst a blister; they usually need no treatment. However, if a blister breaks or is likely to burst, cover it with a nonadhesive sterile dressing that extends well beyond the edges of the blister. Leave the dressing in place until the blister subsides.

Small, superficial burns and scalds are often due to domestic incidents, such as touching a hot iron or oven rack. Most minor burns can be treated successfully by first aid and will heal naturally. However, you should advise the casualty to seek medical advice if you are at all concerned about the severity of the injury (Assessing a burn, pp.172–73).

After a burn, blisters may form. These thin "bubbles" are caused by tissue fluid leaking into the burned area just beneath the skin's surface. You should never break a blister caused by a burn because you may introduce infection into the wound.

WHAT TO DO

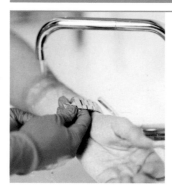

1 **Flood the injured part** with cold water for at least ten minutes or until the pain is relieved. If water is not available, any cold, harmless liquid, such as milk, can be used.

2 **Gently remove any jewelry,** watches, belts, or constricting clothing from the injured area before it begins to swell.

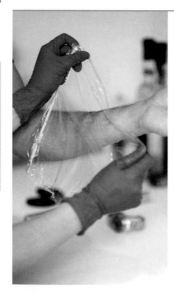

3 **When the burn is cooled,** cover it with plastic wrap or place a clean plastic bag over a foot or hand. Apply the wrap lengthwise over the burn, not around the limb because the tissues swell. If you do not have plastic wrap or a plastic bag, use a sterile dressing or a gauze pad, bandaged loosely in place.

4 **Take or send the casualty** to the hospital if the casualty is a child, or if you are in any doubt about the casualty's condition.

BURNS TO THE AIRWAY

Any burn to the face, mouth, or throat is very serious because the air passages may become swollen. Usually, signs of burning, such as soot or singed nasal hairs, is evident. Suspect damage to the airway if a casualty sustains burns in a confined space—he is likely to have inhaled hot air or gases.

There is no specific first aid treatment for an extreme case of burns to the airway; the swelling will rapidly block the airway, and there is a serious risk of hypoxia. Immediate and specialized medical help is required.

WHAT TO DO

1 **Call 911 for emergency help.** Tell the dispatcher that you suspect burns to the casualty's airway.

2 **Take any steps possible** to improve the casualty's air supply, such as loosening clothing around his neck.

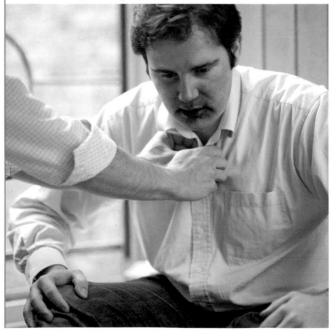

3 **Offer the casualty ice** or small sips of cold water to reduce swelling and pain.

4 **Reassure the casualty.** Monitor and record vital signs—level of response, breathing, and pulse (pp.52–53)—while waiting for help to arrive.

CAUTION
- If the casualty loses consciousness, open the airway and check breathing (The unconscious casualty pp.54–87).

RECOGNITION
There may be:
- Soot around the nose or mouth
- Singeing of the nasal hairs
- Redness, swelling, or actual burning of the tongue
- Damage to the skin around the mouth
- Hoarseness of the voice
- Breathing difficulties

YOUR AIMS
- To maintain an open airway
- To arrange urgent removal to the hospital

ELECTRICAL BURN

RECOGNITION

There may be:

- Unconsciousness
- Full-thickness burns, with swelling, scorching, and charring
- Burns at points of entry and exit of electricity
- Signs of shock (pp.112–13)

YOUR AIMS

- To treat the burns and shock
- To arrange urgent removal to the hospital

Burns may occur when electricity passes through the body. There may be surface damage along the point of contact, or at the points of entry and exit of the current. In addition, there may also be internal damage between the entry and exit points; the position and direction of wounds will alert you to the likely site and extent of hidden injury.

Burns may be caused by a lightning strike or by a low- or high-voltage electric current. Electric shock can cause cardiac arrest. If the casualty is unconscious, your priority, once the area is safe, is to open his airway and check his breathing, and begin CPR immediately if needed.

WHAT TO DO

 1 **Make sure that contact** with the electrical source is broken before you touch the casualty (pp.34–35).

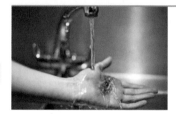 **2** **Flood the injury** with cold water (at the entry and exit points if both are present) for at least ten minutes or until pain is relieved. If water is not available, any cold, harmless liquid can be used.

3 **Gently remove any jewelry,** watches, belts, or constricting clothing from the injured area before it begins to swell. Do not touch the burn.

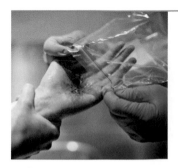 **4** **When the burn is cooled,** place a clean plastic bag over a burn on a foot or hand, taping the bag loosely in place (attach tape to the bag, not the skin). Or, cover the burn with plastic wrap, laying it along the length of the limb so that it does not become too tight. If neither is available, use a sterile dressing or a clean gauze pad loosely.

5 **Call 911 for emergency help.** Reassure the casualty and treat him for shock (pp.112–13). Monitor and record vital signs—level of response, breathing and pulse (pp.52–53)—while waiting for help to arrive.

SEE ALSO Electrical incidents **pp.34–35** | Severe burns and scalds **pp.174–75** | Shock **pp.112–13** | The unconscious casualty **pp.54–87**

CHEMICAL BURN

Certain chemicals may irritate, burn, or penetrate the skin, causing widespread and sometimes fatal damage. Most strong, corrosive chemicals are found in industry, but chemical burns can also occur in the home; for instance from dishwasher products (the most common cause of alkali burns in children), oven cleaners, pesticides, and paint stripper.

Chemical burns are always serious, and the casualty will need urgent hospital treatment. If possible, note the name or brand of the burning substance. Before treating the casualty, ensure the safety of yourself and others because some chemicals give off poisonous fumes, causing breathing difficulties.

WHAT TO DO

1 Make sure that the area around the casualty is safe. Ventilate the area to disperse fumes. Wear protective gloves to prevent you from coming into contact with the chemical. If it is safe to do so, seal the chemical container. Move the casualty if necessary. If the chemical is in powder form, it can be brushed off the skin.

2 Flood the burn with water for at least 20 minutes to disperse the chemical and stop the burning. If treating a casualty lying on the ground, ensure that the contaminated water does not collect underneath her. Pour water away from yourself to avoid being splashed.

RECOGNITION

There may be:
- Evidence of chemicals in the vicinity
- Intense, stinging pain

Later:
- Discoloration, blistering, and peeling
- Swelling of the affected area

YOUR AIMS

- To make the area safe and inform the relevant authority
- To disperse the harmful chemical
- To arrange transportation to the hospital

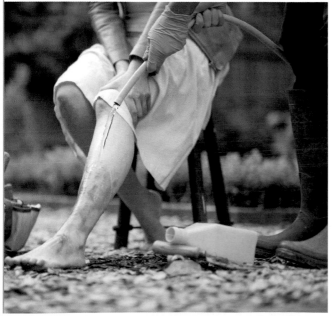

3 Gently remove any contaminated clothing while flooding the injury.

4 Arrange to take or send the casualty to the hospital. Monitor vital signs—level of response, breathing, and pulse (pp.52–53)—while waiting for medical help. Pass on details of the chemical to medical staff if you can identify it.

SEE ALSO Chemical burn to the eye **p.180** | Inhalation of fumes **pp.98–99**

CHEMICAL BURN TO THE EYE

CAUTION

- Do not allow the casualty to touch the injured eye.
- Remove a contact lens only if it slips out easily.
- If the incident occurs in the workplace, notify the safety officer and/or emergency services.

Splashes of chemicals in the eye can cause serious injury if not treated quickly. Some chemicals damage the surface of the eye, resulting in scarring and even blindness.

Your priority is to wash out (irrigate) the eye so that the chemical is diluted and dispersed. When irrigating the eye, be careful that the contaminated rinsing water does not splash you or the casualty. Before beginning to treat the casualty, put on protective gloves if available.

RECOGNITION

There may be:

- Intense pain in the eye
- Inability to open the injured eye
- Redness and swelling around the eye
- Copious watering of the eye
- Evidence of chemical substances or containers in the immediate area

YOUR AIMS

- To disperse the harmful chemical
- To arrange transportation to the hospital

WHAT TO DO

1 **Put on protective gloves.** Hold the casualty's affected eye under gently running cold water for at least ten minutes. Irrigate the eyelid thoroughly both inside and out; if the casualty's eye is shut in a spasm of pain, gently, but firmly, try to pull the eyelid open.

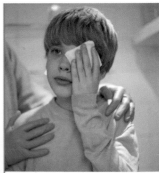

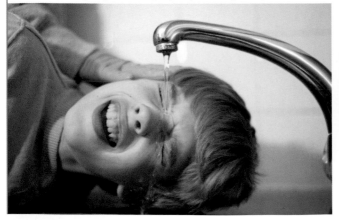

3 Ask the casualty to hold a clean gauze pad over the injured eye. If it will be some time before the casualty receives medical attention, bandage the pad loosely in position.

2 **Make sure that contaminated water** does not splash the uninjured eye. You may find it easier to pour the water over the eye using an eye irrigator or a glass.

4 **Arrange to take or send** the casualty to the hospital. Identify the chemical if possible and pass on details to the medical staff.

FLASH BURN TO THE EYE

This condition occurs when the surface (cornea) of the eye is damaged by exposure to ultraviolet light, such as prolonged glare from sunlight reflected off snow. Symptoms usually develop gradually, and recovery can take up to a week. Flash burns can also be caused by glare from a welder's torch.

CAUTION

- Do not remove the casualty's contact lenses.

WHAT TO DO

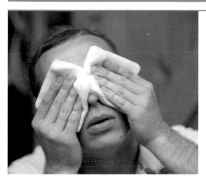

1 **Reassure the casualty.** Ask him to hold an eye pad against each injured eye. If it is likely to take some time to obtain medical attention, lightly bandage the pad(s) in place.

2 **Arrange to take** or send the casualty to the hospital.

RECOGNITION

- Intense pain in the affected eye(s)

There may also be:

- A "gritty" feeling in the eye(s)
- Sensitivity to light
- Redness and watering of the eye(s)

YOUR AIMS

- To prevent further damage
- To arrange transportation to the hospital

INCAPACITANT SPRAY EXPOSURE

There are two types of incapacitant spray—CS spray and pepper spray. Both sprays are used by police forces for riot control and self-protection, and both have been used by unauthorized people as weapons in assault situations. They are both aerosols and have the same effects. The effects usually wear off 15–20 minutes after a person has been exposed to the spray.

CAUTION

- If the casualty suffers from asthma, the spray may trigger an attack.
- If the casualty's symptoms persist, seek medical advice.

WHAT TO DO

1 **Move the casualty** to a well-ventilated area with a free flow of air to ensure rapid dispersal of the spray.

2 **Put on gloves** if you are handling contaminated items such as clothing. Advise the casualty to remove contact lenses—he may need help. Remove wet clothing and put it in a sealed plastic bag.

3 **If necessary,** the casualty may wash his skin with soap and water, paying particular attention to skin folds and ears. Showering may release spray particles trapped in the hair and cause transient irritation.

RECOGNITION

There may be:

- Burning sensation and watering of the eyes
- Sneezing and runny nose
- Stinging sensation on the skin with redness and possibly blistering
- Difficulty breathing

YOUR AIM

- To remove the casualty from the spray area

SEE ALSO Allergy p.222 | Asthma p.102

DEHYDRATION

There may be:

- Dry mouth and dry eyes
- Dry and/or cracked lips
- Headaches (light-headedness)
- Dizziness and confusion
- Dark urine
- Reduction in the amount of urine passed
- Cramp, with a feeling of tightness in the most used muscles, such as the calves
- In babies and young children, pale skin with sunken eyes. In young babies the soft spot on the head (the fontanelle) may be sunken

YOUR AIM

- To replace the lost body fluids and salts

This condition occurs when the amount of fluids lost from the body is not adequately replaced. Dehydration can begin to develop when a person loses as little as one percent of his body weight through fluid loss. A loss of two to six percent of his body weight can occur during a typical period of exercise on a warm day. The average daily intake of fluids is 4 pints (2.5 liters); this fluid loss needs to be replaced. In addition to fluid, the body loses essential body salts through sweating.

Dehydration is primarily the result of: excessive sweating during sporting activities, especially in hot weather; prolonged exposure to sun, or hot, humid conditions; sweating through raised body temperature during a fever; and loss of fluid through severe diarrhea and vomiting. Young children, older people, or those involved in prolonged periods of activity are particularly at risk. Severe dehydration can cause muscle cramps through the loss of body salts.

The aim of first aid is to replace the lost water and salts through rehydration. Water is usually sufficient but oral rehydration solutions can help replace lost salt.

WHAT TO DO

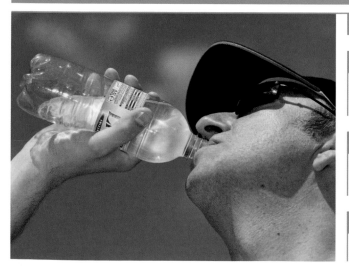

1 Reassure the casualty. Help him sit down.

2 Give him plenty of fluids to drink. Water is usually sufficient but oral rehydration solutions can help with salt replacement.

3 If the casualty is suffering from a cramp, stretch and massage the affected muscles (p.167). Advise the casualty to rest.

4 Monitor and record the casualty's condition. If he remains unwell, seek medical advice right away.

SUNBURN

Overexposure to the sun or a sunlamp can result in sunburn. At high altitudes, sunburn can occur even on an overcast summer's day, or in the snow. Some medicines can trigger severe sensitivity to sunlight. Rarely, skin burns can be caused by exposure to radioactivity.

Sunburn can be prevented by staying in the shade, wearing protective clothing, and regularly applying high sun protection factor sunscreen or sun block.

Most sunburn is superficial; in severe cases, the skin is lobster-red and blistered. In addition, the casualty may suffer from heat exhaustion or heatstroke.

RECOGNITION

■ Reddened skin
■ Pain in the area of the burn

Later there may be:

■ Blistering of the affected skin

YOUR AIMS

■ To move the casualty out of the sun as soon as possible
■ To relieve discomfort and pain

WHAT TO DO

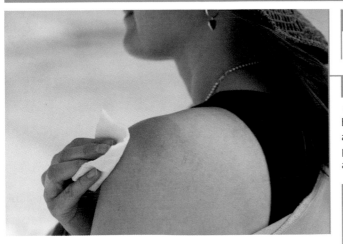

1 Cover the casualty's skin with light clothing or a towel. Help her move out of the sun or, if at all possible, indoors.

2 Encourage the casualty to have frequent sips of cold water. Cool the affected skin by dabbing with cold water. If the area is extensive, the casualty may prefer to soak the affected skin in a cold bath for ten minutes.

3 If the burns are mild, calamine or an after-sun lotion may soothe them. Advise the casualty to stay inside or in the shade. If sunburn is severe, seek medical advice.

SEE ALSO Dehydration **opposite** | Heat exhaustion **p.184** | Heatstroke **p.185** | Minor burns and scalds **p.176** | **183**

HEAT EXHAUSTION

RECOGNITION

As the condition develops, there may be:

- Headache, dizziness, and confusion
- Loss of appetite and nausea
- Sweating, with pale, clammy skin
- Cramps in the arms, legs, or abdomen
- Rapid, weakening pulse and breathing

YOUR AIMS

- To cool the casualty down
- To replace lost body fluids and salts
- To obtain medical help if necessary

This disorder is caused by loss of salt and water from the body through excessive sweating. It usually develops gradually and often affects people who are not acclimatized to hot, humid conditions. People who are unwell, especially those with illnesses that cause vomiting and diarrhea, are more susceptible than others to developing heat exhaustion.

A dangerous and common cause of heat exhaustion occurs when the body produces more heat than it can cope with. Some nonprescription drugs, such as ecstasy, can affect the body's temperature regulation system. This, combined with the exertion of dancing in a warm environment, can result in a person becoming overheated and dehydrated. These effects can lead to heatstroke and even death.

WHAT TO DO

1 **Help the casualty to a cool,** shady place. Get him to lie down and raise and support his legs to improve blood flow to his brain.

2 **Give him plenty of water to drink.** Oral rehydration salts or isotonic drinks will help with salt replacement.

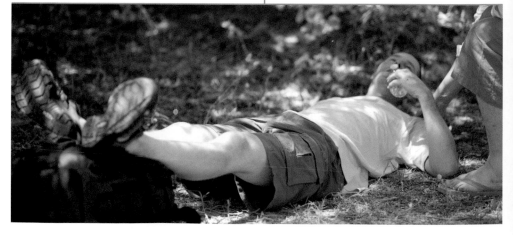

3 **Monitor and record vital signs**—level of response, breathing, and pulse (pp.52–53). Even if the casualty recovers quickly, advise him to seek medical help.

4 If the casualty's vital signs worsen, **call 911 for emergency help.** Monitor and record vital signs—level of response, breathing, and pulse (pp.52–53)—while you are waiting for help to arrive.

HEATSTROKE

A medical emergency, this condition is caused by a failure of the "thermostat" in the brain to regulate body temperature. The body becomes dangerously overheated, usually due to a high fever or prolonged exposure to heat. Heatstroke can also result from the use of drugs such as ecstasy. In some cases, heatstroke follows heat exhaustion when sweating ceases and the body cannot be cooled by the evaporation of sweat.

Heatstroke can develop with little warning, resulting in unconsciousness within minutes of the casualty feeling unwell.

WHAT TO DO

1 Quickly move the casualty to a cool place. Remove as much of his outer clothing as possible. **Call 911 for emergency help.**

2 While waiting for emergency help, assist the casualty to sit down, supported with cushions. The best way to cool the casualty is to spray him with water and then fan him, repeatedly. A cold, wet sheet may also work, and ice packs in the armpits and groin may be affective.

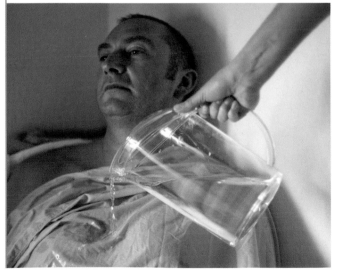

3 Once the casualty's temperature appears to have returned to normal, replace the wet sheet with a dry one.

4 Monitor and record vital signs—level of response, breathing, pulse, and temperature (pp.52–53)—while waiting for help. If the casualty's temperature rises again, repeat the cooling process.

CAUTION
- If the casualty loses consciousness, and is not breathing (or is just gasping), begin CPR with chest compressions (pp.54–87).

RECOGNITION
There may be:
- Headache, dizziness, and discomfort
- Restlessness and confusion
- Hot, flushed, and dry skin
- Rapid deterioration in the level of response
- Full, bounding pulse
- Body temperature above 104°F (40°C)

YOUR AIMS
- To lower the casualty's body temperature as quickly as possible
- To arrange urgent removal to the hospital

HYPOTHERMIA

RECOGNITION

As hypothermia develops, there may be:

- Shivering, and cold, pale, dry skin
- Apathy, disorientation, or irrational behavior
- Lethargy or impaired consciousness
- Slow and shallow breathing
- Slow and weakening pulse. In extreme cases, the heart may stop

YOUR AIMS

- To prevent the casualty from losing more body heat
- To rewarm the casualty quickly
- To obtain emergency help if necessary

This condition develops when the body temperature falls below 95°F (35°C). The effects vary depending on the speed of onset and the level to which the body temperature falls. The blood supply to the superficial blood vessels in the skin, for example, shuts down to maintain the function of the vital organs such as the heart and brain. Moderate hypothermia can usually be reversed. Severe hypothermia—when the core body temperature falls below 86°F (30°C)—is often, although not always, fatal. No matter how low the body temperature becomes, persist with life-saving procedures until emergency help arrives because in cases of hypothermia, survival may be possible even after prolonged periods of resuscitation.

WHAT CAUSES HYPOTHERMIA

Hypothermia can be caused by prolonged exposure to cold. Moving air has a much greater cooling effect than still air, so a high "wind-chill factor" in cold weather can substantially increase the risk of a person developing hypothermia. Immersion in cold water can cause death from hypothermia. When surrounded by cold water, the body can cool up to 30 times faster than in dry air, and body temperature falls rapidly.

Hypothermia may also develop indoors in poorly heated houses. Elderly people, infants, homeless people, and those who are thin and frail are particularly vulnerable. Lack of activity, chronic illness and fatigue all increase the risk; alcohol and drugs can exacerbate the condition.

TREATMENT WHEN OUTDOORS

1 **Take the casualty** to a sheltered place as quickly as possible. Shield the casualty from the wind.

2 **Remove and replace** any wet clothing if possible; do not give him your clothes. Make sure his head is covered.

3 **Protect the casualty** from the ground. Lay him on a thick layer of dry insulating material, such as pine branches. Put him in a dry sleeping bag and/or cover him with blankets or newspapers. Wrap him in a plastic or foil survival bag, if available. You can shelter and warm him with your body.

4 **Call 911 or send for emergency help.** Ideally, two people should go for help and stay together if you are in a remote area. It is important that you do not leave the casualty by himself; someone must remain with him at all times.

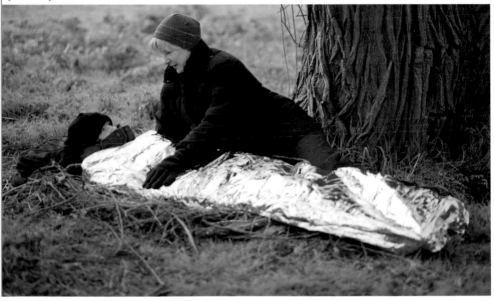

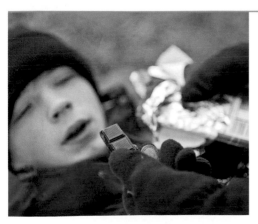

5 **To help rewarm a casualty** who is conscious, give him warm drinks and high-energy foods such as chocolate, if available.

6 Monitor and record the casualty's vital signs—level of response, breathing, pulse, and temperature (pp.52–53)—while waiting for help to arrive.

≪ HYPOTHERMIA

TREATMENT WHEN INDOORS

1 The casualty must be rewarmed quickly. Cover him with layers of blankets and warm the room to about 77°F (25°C).

2 Give the casualty a warm drink such as soup and/or high-energy foods such as chocolate to help rewarm him.

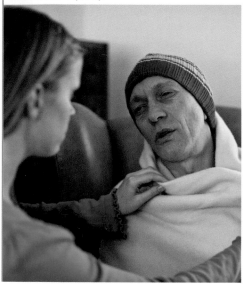

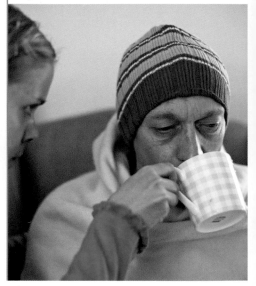

3 Seek medical advice. Be aware that in the elderly, hypothermia may also be disguising the symptoms of a stroke (pp.212–13), a heart attack (p.211), an underactive thyroid gland (hypothyroidism), or a severe infection.

4 Monitor and record the casualty's vital signs—level of response, breathing, pulse, and temperature (pp.52–53)—as he is rewarmed.

SPECIAL CASE HYPOTHERMIA IN INFANTS

A baby's mechanisms for regulating body temperature are underdeveloped, so she may develop hypothermia in a cold room. The baby's skin may look healthy but feel cold, and she may be limp and unusually quiet, and refuse to feed. Rewarm a cold baby by wrapping her in blankets and warming the room. You should always seek medical advice if you suspect a baby has hypothermia.

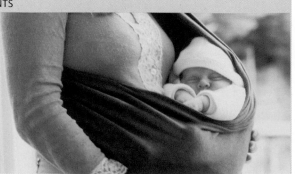

FROSTBITE

With this condition, the tissues of the extremities—usually the fingers and toes—freeze due to low temperatures. In severe cases, this freezing can lead to permanent loss of sensation and, eventually, tissue death and gangrene as the blood vessels and soft tissues become permanently damaged.

Frostbite usually occurs in freezing or cold and windy conditions. People who cannot move around to increase their circulation are particularly susceptible.

In many cases, frostbite is accompanied by hypothermia (pp.186–87), and this should be treated accordingly.

WHAT TO DO

1 **Advise the casualty** to put his hands, if affected, in his armpits. Move the casualty into warmth before you thaw the affected part further.

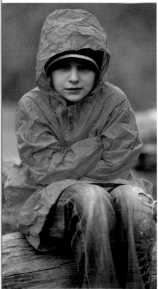

2 **Once inside,** gently remove gloves, rings, and any other constrictions, such as boots. Warm the affected part with your hands, in your lap, or continue to warm them in the casualty's armpits. Avoid rubbing the affected area because this can damage skin and other tissues.

3 **Place the affected parts** in tepid water, or lower than 104°F (40°C). Dry gently and apply a light dressing of dry gauze bandage.

4 **Raise the affected** limb to reduce swelling. An adult may take the recommended dose of acetaminophen, or her own pain medicine, and a child, the recommended dose of acetaminophen syrup (not aspirin). Take or send the casualty to the hospital.

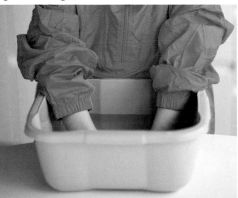

CAUTION

- Do not put the affected part near direct heat.
- Do not attempt to thaw the affected part until there is no danger of it refreezing.

RECOGNITION

There may be:

- At first, "pins-and-needles"
- Paleness (pallor) followed by numbness
- Hardening and stiffening of the skin
- A color change of the skin of the affected area: first white, then mottled and blue. On recovery, the skin may be red, hot, painful, and blistered. Where gangrene occurs, the tissue may become black due to loss of blood supply.

YOUR AIMS

- To warm the affected area slowly to prevent further tissue damage
- To arrange transportation to the hospital

SEE ALSO Hypothermia pp.186–88 | **189**

9

Objects that find their way into the body, either through a wound in the skin or via an orifice, are known as "foreign bodies." These range from grit in eye to small objects that young children may push into their noses and ears. These can be distressing but do not usually cause serious problems for the casualty.

Poisoning may result from exposure to or ingestion of toxic substances, chemicals, and contaminated food. The effects of poisons vary but medical advice will be needed in most cases.

Insect stings and marine stings can often be treated with first aid. However, multiple stings can produce a reaction that requires urgent medical help. Animal and human bites always require medical attention due to the risk of infection.

AIMS AND OBJECTIVES

- To ensure the safety of yourself and the casualty
- To assess the casualty's condition quickly and calmly
- To assess the potential danger of a foreign object
- To identify the poisonous substance
- To comfort and reassure the casualty
- To look for and treat any injuries associated with the condition
- To obtain medical help if necessary. **Call 911 for emergency help** if you suspect a serious illness or injury, or anaphylaxis
- To be aware of your own needs

FOREIGN OBJECTS, POISONING, BITES & STINGS

THE SENSORY ORGANS

THE SKIN

The body is covered and protected by the skin. This is one of the body's largest organs and is made up of two layers: the outer layer, called the epidermis, and an inner layer, the dermis. The skin forms a barrier against harmful substances and germs. It is also an important sense organ, containing nerves that ensure that the body is sensitive to heat, cold, pain, and touch.

Structure of the skin

The skin consists of the thin epidermis and the thicker dermis, which sit on a layer of fatty tissue (subcutaneous fat). Blood vessels, nerves, muscles, sebaceous (oil) glands, sweat glands, and hair roots (follicles) lie in the dermis.

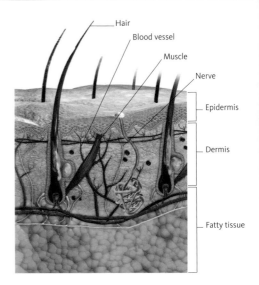

Hair
Blood vessel
Muscle
Nerve
Epidermis
Dermis
Fatty tissue

THE EYES

These complex organs enable us to see the world around us. Each eye consists of a colored part (iris) with a small opening (pupil) that allows light to enter the eye. The size of the pupil changes according to the amount of light that is entering the eye.

Light is focused by the transparent lens onto a "screen" (retina) at the back of the eye. Special cells in the retina convert this information into electrical impulses that then travel, via the optic nerve that leads from the eye, to the part of the brain where the impulses are analyzed.

Each eye is protected by a bony socket in the skull (p.133). The eyelids and delicate membranes called conjunctiva protect the front of the eyes.

Tears form a protective film across the front of the conjunctiva, lubricating the surface and flushing away dust and dirt.

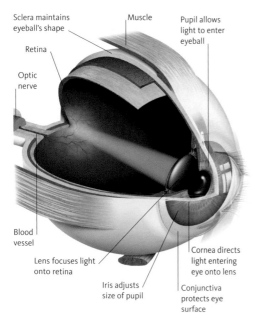

Sclera maintains eyeball's shape
Muscle
Pupil allows light to enter eyeball
Retina
Optic nerve
Blood vessel
Lens focuses light onto retina
Iris adjusts size of pupil
Cornea directs light entering eye onto lens
Conjunctiva protects eye surface

Structure of the eye

The eyes are fluid-filled, spherical structures about 1 in (2.5 cm) in diameter. They have focusing parts (cornea and lens), and light- and color-sensitive cells in the retina.

THE EARS

In addition to being the organs of hearing, the ears play an important role in balance. The visible part of each ear, the auricle, funnels sounds into the ear canal to vibrate the eardrum. Fine hairs in the ear canal filter out dust, and glands secrete ear wax to trap any other small particles. The vibrations of the eardrum pass across the middle ear to the hearing apparatus (cochlea) in the inner ear. This structure converts the vibrations into nerve impulses and transmits them to the brain via the auditory nerve. The vestibular apparatus within the inner ear is involved in balance.

Structure of the ear

The ear is divided into three main parts: the outer, middle, and inner ear. The eardrum separates the outer and middle ear. The inner ear contains the organs of hearing and balance.

Scalp muscle

Auricular cartilage

Eardrum vibrates in response to sound

Vestibular apparatus regulates balance

Auditory nerve transmits sound impulses to brain

Cochlea contains receptor for hearing

Ear canal

Eustachian tube connects middle ear with back of nose and throat

Pinna (ear flap)

Outer ear   Middle ear   Inner ear

THE MOUTH AND NOSE

These cavities form the entrances to the digestive and respiratory tracts respectively. The nasal cavities connect with the throat. They are lined with blood vessels and membranes that secrete mucus to trap debris as it enters the nose. Food enters the digestive tract via the mouth, which leads into the esophagus. The epiglottis, a flap at the back of the throat, prevents food from entering the windpipe (trachea).

Structure of the mouth and nose

The nostrils lead into the two nasal cavities, which are lined with mucous membranes and blood vessels. The nasal cavities connect directly with the top of the throat, which is at the back of the mouth.

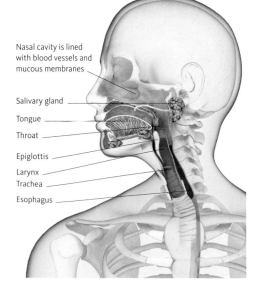

Nasal cavity is lined with blood vessels and mucous membranes

Salivary gland

Tongue

Throat

Epiglottis

Larynx

Trachea

Esophagus

SPLINTER

Small splinters of wood, metal, or glass may enter the skin. They carry a risk of infection because they are rarely clean. Often a splinter can be successfully withdrawn from the skin using tweezers. However, if the splinter is deeply embedded, lies over a joint, or is difficult to remove, you should leave it in place and advise the casualty to seek medical help.

YOUR AIMS

- To remove the splinter
- To minimize the risk of infection

SPECIAL CASE EMBEDDED SPLINTER

If a splinter is embedded or difficult to dislodge, do not probe the area with a sharp object, such as a needle, or you may introduce infection. Pad around the splinter until you can bandage over it without pressing on it, and seek medical help.

WHAT TO DO

1 **Gently clean the area** around the splinter with soap and warm water.

2 **Hold the tweezers** close to the end for a better grip. Grasp the splinter with tweezers as close to the skin as possible.

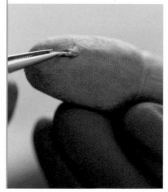

3 **Draw the splinter** out in a straight line at the same angle that it went into the skin; make sure it does not break.

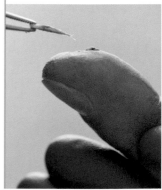

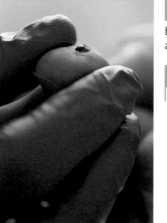

4 **Carefully squeeze** the wound to encourage a little bleeding. This will help flush out any remaining dirt.

5 **Wash again** with soap and water. Clean and dry the wound and cover with a dressing.

EMBEDDED FISHHOOK

A fishhook that is embedded in the skin is difficult to remove because of the barb at the end of the hook. If possible, you should ensure that the hook is removed by a healthcare professional. Only attempt to remove a hook yourself if medical help is not readily available. Embedded fishhooks carry a risk of infection, including tetanus.

CAUTION

- Do not try to pull out a fishhook unless you can cut off the barb. If you cannot, seek medical help.
- Seek medical advice if he is not sure if he is up to date on his tetanus immunization.

WHAT TO DO

1 Support the injured area. If possible, cut off the fishing line as close to the hook as possible.

2 If medical help is readily available, build up pads of gauze around the hook until you can bandage over the top without pushing it in farther. Bandage over the padding and the hook and arrange to take or send the casualty to the hospital.

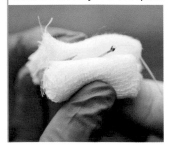

3 If medical help is unavailable, you can try to remove the hook if you can see the barb. Cut off the barb with wirecutters, then carefully withdraw the hook back through the skin by its eye.

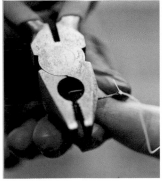

4 **Clean and dry** the wound and cover with a dressing.

YOUR AIMS

- To obtain medical help
- To minimize the risk of infection
- If help is delayed, to remove the fishhook without causing the casualty any further injury and pain

SWALLOWED FOREIGN OBJECT

Children may put small items in their mouths when playing. An adult may swallow a bone by mistake or ingest unlikely objects on purpose. Most objects will pass through the digestive system, but some can cause a blockage or perforation.

CAUTION

- Do not let the casualty make himself vomit because the object could damage the esophagus.

WHAT TO DO

1 **Reassure the casualty** and find out what he swallowed.

2 **Seek medical advice.**

YOUR AIM

- To obtain medical advice as soon as possible

FOREIGN OBJECT IN THE EYE

Foreign objects such as grit, a loose eyelash, or a contact lens that are floating on the surface of the eye can be easily rinsed out. However, you must not attempt to remove anything that sticks to the eye or penetrates the eyeball because this may damage the eye. Instead, make sure that the casualty receives urgent medical attention.

RECOGNITION

There may be:

- Blurred vision
- Pain or discomfort
- Redness and watering of the eye
- Eyelids held tight in spasm

YOUR AIM

- To prevent injury to the eye

SPECIAL CASE IF OBJECT IS UNDER UPPER EYELID

Ask the casualty to grasp the lashes on her upper eyelid and pull the upper lid over the lower lid; the lower lashes may brush the particle clear. If this is unsuccessful, ask her to try blinking underwater because this may also make the object float off. Do not attempt to do this if the object is large or abrasive.

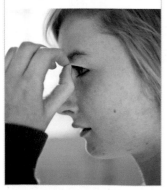

WHAT TO DO

1 **Advise the casualty** not to rub her eye. Ask her to sit down facing a light.

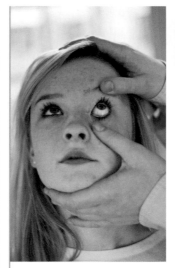 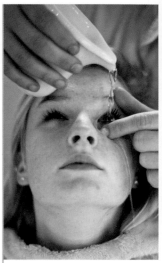

2 **Stand beside,** or just behind, the casualty. Gently separate her eyelids with your thumbs or finger and thumb. Ask her to look right, left, up, and down. Examine every part of her eye as she does this.

3 **If you can see a foreign object** on the white of the eye, wash it out by pouring clean water from a glass or pitcher, or by using a sterile eyewash if you have one. Put a towel around the casualty's shoulders. Hold her eye open and pour the water from the inner corner so that it drains onto the towel.

4 **If this is unsuccessful,** try lifting the object off with a moist swab or the damp corner of a clean handkerchief or tissue. If you still cannot remove the object, seek medical help.

FOREIGN OBJECT IN THE EAR

If a foreign object becomes lodged in the ear, it may cause temporary loss of hearing by blocking the ear canal. In some cases, a foreign object may damage the eardrum. Young children frequently push objects into their ears. The tips of cotton swabs are often left in the ear. Insects can fly or crawl into the ear and may cause distress.

WHAT TO DO

1 Arrange to take or send the casualty to the hospital. Do not try to remove a lodged foreign object yourself.

2 Reassure the casualty during the journey or until medical help arrives.

YOUR AIMS

- To prevent injury to the ear
- To remove a trapped insect
- To arrange transportation to the hospital if a foreign object is lodged in the ear

SPECIAL CASE INSECT INSIDE THE EAR

Reassure the casualty and ask him to sit down. Support his head, with the affected ear uppermost. Gently flood the ear with tepid water; the insect should float out. If this flooding does not remove the insect, seek medical help.

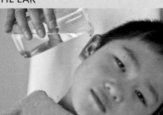

FOREIGN OBJECT IN THE NOSE

Young children may push small objects up their noses. Objects can block the nose and cause infection. If the object is sharp it can damage the tissues, and "button" batteries can cause burns and bleeding. Do not try to remove a foreign object; you may cause injury or push it farther into the airway.

WHAT TO DO

1 Try to keep the casualty quiet and calm. Tell him to breathe through his mouth at a normal rate. Advise him not to poke inside his nose to try to remove the object himself.

2 Arrange to take or send the casualty to the hospital, so that it can be safely removed by medical staff.

RECOGNITION

There may be:

- Difficult or noisy breathing through the nose
- Swelling of the nose
- Smelly or blood-stained discharge, indicating that an object may have been lodged for some time

YOUR AIM

- To arrange transportation to the hospital

HOW POISONS AFFECT THE BODY

A poison (toxin) is a substance that, if taken into or absorbed into the body in sufficient quantity, can cause either temporary or permanent damage.

Poisons can be swallowed, absorbed through the skin, inhaled, splashed into the eyes, or injected. Once in the body, they may enter the bloodstream and be carried swiftly to all organs and tissues. Signs and symptoms of poisoning vary with the poison. They may develop quickly or over a number of days. Vomiting is common, especially when the poison has been ingested. Inhaled poisons often cause breathing difficulties.

Effects of poisons on the body
Poisons can enter the body through the skin, digestive system, lungs, or bloodstream. Once there, they can be carried to all parts of the body and cause multiple side effects.

Poisons reaching the brain may cause confusion, delirium, seizures, and unconsciousness

Swallowed corrosive chemicals can burn the mouth, lips, and food passage (esophagus)

Poisonous gases, solvents, vapors, or fumes can be inhaled and affect the airways and lungs, causing severe breathing problems

Poisons can seriously damage the liver

Poisons in the digestive system can cause vomiting, abdominal pain, and diarrhea

Corrosive chemicals can burn the skin. Pesticides and plant toxins may be absorbed through the skin, causing local or general reactions

Injected poisons and drugs rapidly enter the bloodstream; some prevent blood cells from carrying oxygen to body tissues

Some poisons disturb the action of the heart by interrupting its normal electrical activity

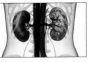

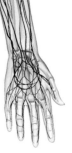

Poisons reaching the kidneys (situated toward the back of the body behind the large intestine) from the bloodstream can cause serious damage to these organs

TYPES OF POISONS

Some poisons are man-made—for example, chemicals and drugs—and these are found in the home as well as in industry. Almost every household contains substances that are potentially poisonous, such as bleach and paint stripper, as well as prescribed or over-the-counter medicines, which may be dangerous if taken in excessive amounts.

Other poisons occur in nature: for example, plants produce poisons that may irritate the skin or cause more serious symptoms if ingested, and various insects and creatures produce venom in their bites and stings. Contamination of food by bacteria may result in food poisoning—one of the most common forms of poisoning.

RECOGNIZING AND TREATING THE EFFECTS OF POISONING

ROUTE OF ENTRY INTO THE BODY	POISON	POSSIBLE EFFECTS	ACTION
Swallowed (ingested)	■ Drugs and alcohol ■ Cleaning products ■ Home improvement and gardening products ■ Plant poisons ■ Bacterial food poisons ■ Viral food poisons	■ Nausea and vomiting ■ Abdominal pain ■ Seizures ■ Irregular, or fast or slow, heartbeat ■ Impaired consciousness	■ Monitor casualty ■ **Call emergency help** ■ Start CPR if necessary (pp.54–87) ■ Use a face mask to protect yourself if you need to give rescue breaths
Absorbed through the skin	■ Cleaning products ■ Home improvement and gardening products ■ Industrial poisons ■ Plant poisons	■ Pain ■ Swelling ■ Rash ■ Redness ■ Itching	■ Remove contaminated clothing ■ Wash with cold water for 20 minutes ■ Seek medical help ■ Start CPR if necessary (pp.54–87)
Inhaled	■ Fumes of cleaning and construction products ■ Industrial poisons ■ Fumes from fires	■ Difficulty breathing ■ Hypoxia ■ Gray-blue skin (cyanosis) ■ Cherry red lips	■ Help casualty into fresh air ■ **Call emergency help** ■ Start CPR if necessary (pp.54–87)
Splashed in the eye	■ Cleaning products ■ Home improvement and gardening products ■ Industrial poisons ■ Plant poisons	■ Pain and watering of the eye ■ Blurred vision	■ Irrigate the eye for ten minutes (p.180) ■ **Call emergency help** ■ Start CPR if necessary (pp.54–87)
Injected through the skin	■ Venom from stings and bites ■ Drugs	■ Pain, redness, and swelling at injection site ■ Blurred vision ■ Nausea and vomiting ■ Difficulty breathing ■ Seizures ■ Impaired consciousness ■ Anaphylactic shock	For sting/venom: ■ Remove sting, if possible ■ **Call emergency help** ■ Start CPR if necessary (pp.54–87) For injected drugs: ■ **Call emergency help** ■ Start CPR if necessary (pp.54–87)

SWALLOWED POISONS

RECOGNITION

- History of ingestion/exposure

Depending on what has been swallowed, there may be:

- Vomiting, sometimes bloodstained, later diarrhea
- Cramping abdominal pains
- Pain or a burning sensation
- Empty containers in the vicinity
- Impaired consciousness
- Seizures

YOUR AIMS

- To maintain an open airway, breathing, and circulation
- To remove any contaminated clothing
- To identify the poison
- To arrange urgent removal to the hospital

Chemicals that are swallowed may harm the digestive tract, or cause more widespread damage if they enter the bloodstream and are transported to other parts of the body. Hazardous chemicals include household substances such as bleach and paint stripper, which are poisonous or corrosive if swallowed. Drugs, both prescribed or those bought over the counter, can also be harmful if an overdose is taken. Some plants and their berries can also be poisonous.

WHAT TO DO

1 **If the casualty is conscious,** ask her what she has swallowed, and if possible how much and when. Look for clues—for example, poisonous plants, berries or empty containers. Try to reassure her.

2 **Call Poison Control Center (800-222-1222).** If the casualty is unconscious, **call 911 for emergency help**. Give the dispatcher as much information as possible about the poison. This information will help the medical team treat the casualty.

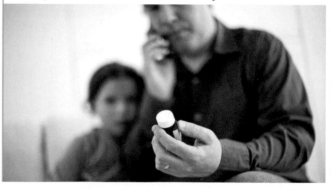

3 **Monitor and record** the casualty's vital signs (pp.52–53) while waiting for help to arrive. Keep samples of any vomited material. Give these samples, containers, and any others clues to the emergency services.

SPECIAL CASE IF LIPS ARE BURNED

If the casualty's lips are burned by corrosive substances, give him frequent sips of cold milk or water while waiting for help to arrive.

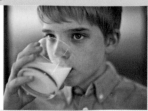

SEE ALSO Alcohol poisoning **p.202** | Chemical burn **p.179** | Drug poisoning **opposite** | Inhalation of fumes **pp.98–99** | The unconscious casualty **pp.54–87**

DRUG POISONING

Poisoning can result from an overdose of prescribed drugs, or drugs that are bought over the counter. It can also be caused by drug abuse or drug interaction. The effects vary depending on the type of drug and how it is taken (below). When you call the emergency services, give as much information as possible. While waiting for help to arrive, look for containers that might help you identify the drug.

WHAT TO DO

1 If the casualty is conscious, help him into a comfortable position and ask him what he has taken. Reassure him while you talk to him.

2 Call 911 for emergency help. Tell the dispatcher you suspect drug poisoning. Monitor and record vital signs—level of response, breathing and pulse (pp.52–53)—while waiting.

3 Keep samples of any vomited material. Look for evidence that might help identify the drug, such as empty containers. Give these samples and containers to the ambulance personnel.

YOUR AIMS

- To maintain breathing and circulation
- To arrange removal to the hospital

RECOGNIZING THE EFFECTS OF DRUG POISONING

CATEGORY	DRUG	EFFECTS OF POISONING
Pain relievers	■ Aspirin (swallowed)	■ Upper abdominal pain, nausea and vomiting ■ Ringing in the ears ■ "Sighing" when breathing ■ Confusion and delirium ■ Dizziness
	■ Acetaminophen (swallowed)	■ Little effect at first, but abdominal pain, nausea, and vomiting may develop ■ Irreversible liver damage may occur within three days (alcohol and malnourishment increase the risk)
Nervous system depressants and tranquilizers	■ Barbiturates and benzodiazepines (swallowed)	■ Lethargy and sleepiness, leading to unconsciousness ■ Shallow breathing ■ Weak, irregular or abnormally slow or fast pulse
Stimulants and hallucinogens	■ Amphetamines (including ecstasy) and LSD (swallowed) ■ Cocaine (inhaled or injected)	■ Excitable, hyperactive behavior, agitation ■ Sweating ■ Tremor of the hands ■ Hallucinations, in which the casualty may claim to "hear voices" or "see things" ■ Dilated pupils
Narcotics	■ Morphine, heroin (commonly injected)	■ Small pupils ■ Sluggishness and confusion, possibly leading to unconsciousness ■ Slow, shallow breathing, which may stop altogether ■ Needle marks, which may be infected
Solvents	■ Glue, lighter fuel (inhaled)	■ Nausea and vomiting ■ Headaches ■ Hallucinations ■ Possibly, unconsciousness ■ Rarely, cardiac arrest
Anesthetic	■ Ketamine	■ Drowsiness ■ Shallow breathing ■ Hallucinations

SEE ALSO The unconscious casualty pp.54–87 |

ALCOHOL POISONING

RECOGNITION

There may be:

- A strong smell of alcohol
- Empty bottles or cans
- Impaired consciousness: the casualty may respond if roused, but will quickly relapse
- Flushed and moist face
- Deep, noisy breathing
- Full, bounding pulse
- Unconsciousness

In the later stages of unconsciousness:

- Shallow breathing
- Weak, rapid pulse
- Dilated pupils that react poorly to light

YOUR AIMS

- To maintain an open airway
- To assess for other conditions
- To seek medical help if necessary

Alcohol is a drug that depresses the activity of the central nervous system—in particular, the brain (pp.142–43). Prolonged or excessive intake of alcohol can severely impair all physical and mental functions, and the person may sink into deep unconsciousness.

There are other risks to a casualty from alcohol poisoning. For example: an unconscious casualty may inhale and choke on vomit; alcohol widens (dilates) the blood vessels so the body loses heat, and hypothermia may develop.

A casualty who smells of alcohol may be misdiagnosed and not receive appropriate treatment for an underlying cause of unconsciousness, such as a head injury, stroke, heart attack, or hypoglycemia.

WHAT TO DO

1 **Cover the casualty with a coat** or blanket to protect him from the cold.

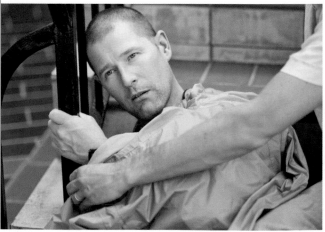

2 **Assess the casualty** for any injuries, especially head injuries, or other medical conditions.

3 **Monitor and record vital signs**—level of response, pulse, and breathing (pp.52–53)—until the casualty recovers or is placed in the care of a responsible person. If you are in any doubt about the casualty's condition, **call 911 for emergency help.**

| **SEE ALSO** Head injury **pp.144–45** | Heart attack **p.211** | Stroke **pp.212–13** | Hypoglycemia **p.215** | Hypothermia **p.186–88** | The unconscious casualty **pp.54–87**

ANIMAL AND HUMAN BITES

Bites from sharp, pointed teeth cause deep puncture wounds that can damage tissues and introduce germs. Bites also crush the tissue. Any bite that breaks the skin needs prompt first aid because there is a high risk of infection.

A serious risk is rabies, a potentially fatal viral infection of the nervous system. The virus is carried in the saliva of infected animals. If bitten in an area where there is a risk of rabies, seek medical advice because the casualty must be given antirabies injections. Try to identify the animal but do not attempt to approach or trap it. Tetanus is also a potential risk following any animal bite.

Human bites carry only a small risk of transmitting the hepatis or HIV/AIDS viruses. However, medical advice should be sought right away.

CAUTION

- If you suspect rabies, arrange to take or send the casualty to the hospital immediately.
- Ask the casualty about tetanus immunization. Seek medical advice if he is unsure if he is up-to-date with his immunizations.

YOUR AIMS

- To control bleeding
- To minimize the risk of infection
- To obtain medical help if necessary

WHAT TO DO

1 Wash the bite wound thoroughly with soap and warm water in order to minimize the risk of infection.

2 Raise and support the wound and pat dry with clean gauze swabs. Then cover with a sterile wound dressing.

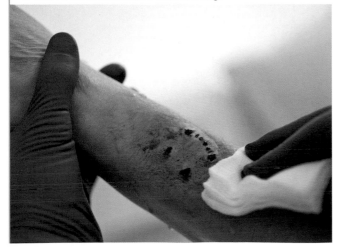

SPECIAL CASE
FOR A DEEP WOUND

If the wound is deep, control bleeding by applying direct pressure over a sterile pad and raise the injured part. Cover the wound and pad with a sterile dressing or large, clean nonfluffy pad and bandage firmly in place. Treat the casualty for shock and **call 911 for emergency help.**

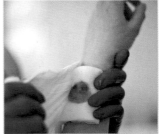

3 Arrange to take or send the casualty to the hospital if the bite breaks the skin; many will require antibiotics.

SEE ALSO Cuts and scrapes **p.119** | Infected wound **p.120** | Severe external bleeding **pp.114–15** | Shock **pp.112–13**

INSECT STING

CAUTION

- **Call 911 for emergency help** if the casualty shows signs of anaphylactic shock (p.223), such as breathing difficulties and/or swelling of the face and neck. Monitor and record vital signs—level of response, breathing, and pulse (pp.52–53)—while waiting for help to arrive.

Usually, a sting from a bee, wasp, or hornet is painful rather than dangerous. An initial sharp pain is followed by mild swelling, redness, and soreness.

However, multiple insect stings can produce a serious reaction. A sting in the mouth or throat is potentially dangerous because swelling can obstruct the airway. With any bite or sting, it is important to watch for signs of an allergic reaction, which can lead to anaphylactic shock (p.223).

RECOGNITION

- Pain at the site of the sting
- Redness and swelling around the site of the sting

YOUR AIMS

- To relieve swelling and pain
- To arrange removal to the hospital if necessary

SPECIAL CASE
STINGS IN THE MOUTH AND THROAT

If a casualty has been stung in the mouth, there is a risk that swelling of tissues in the mouth and/or throat may occur, causing the airway to become blocked. To help prevent this, give the casualty an ice cube to suck or a glass of cold water to sip. **Call 911 for emergency help** if swelling starts to develop.

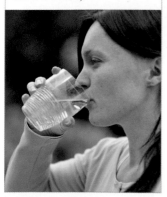

WHAT TO DO

1 **Reassure the casualty.** If the sting is visible, brush or scrape it off sideways with the edge of a credit card or your fingernail. Do not use tweezers because you could squeeze the stinger and inject more poison into the casualty.

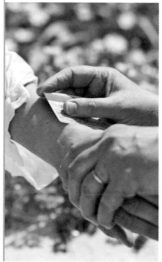

2 **Raise the affected part** if possible, and apply a cold compress such as an ice pack (p.241) to minimize swelling. Advise the casualty to keep the compress in place for at least ten minutes. Tell her to seek medical advice if the pain and swelling persist.

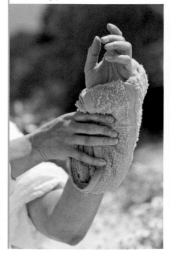

3 **Monitor vital signs**—level of response, breathing, and pulse (pp.52–53). Watch for signs of an allergic reaction, such as wheezing and/or reddened, swollen, itchy skin.

TICK BITE

Ticks are tiny, spiderlike creatures found in grass or woodlands. They attach themselves to passing animals (including humans) and bite into the skin to suck blood. When sucking blood, a tick swells to about the size of a pea, and it can then be seen easily. Ticks can carry disease and cause infection, so they should be removed as soon as possible.

CAUTION
- Do not try to remove the tick with butter or petroleum jelly or burn or freeze it, since it may regurgitate infective fluids into the casualty.

WHAT TO DO

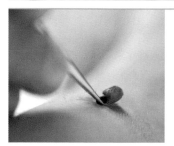

1 Using tweezers, grasp the tick's head as close to the casualty's skin as you can. Gently pull the head upward using steady, even pressure. Do not jerk the tick, which may leave the mouth parts embedded or cause the tick to regurgitate infective fluids into the skin.

YOUR AIM
- To remove the tick

2 Save the tick for identification; place it in a sealed plastic bag. The casualty should seek medical advice; tell him to take the tick because it may be required for analysis.

OTHER BITES AND STINGS

Scorpion stings as well as bites from some spiders and mosquitoes can cause serious illness, and may be fatal.

Bites or stings in the mouth or throat are potentially dangerous because swelling can obstruct the airway. Be alert to an allergic reaction, which may lead the casualty to suffer anaphylactic shock (p.223).

CAUTION
- **Call 911 for emergency help** if a scorpion or a black widow spider has stung the casualty, or if he is showing signs of anaphylactic shock (p.223).

WHAT TO DO

1 Reassure the casualty and help him sit or lie down.

2 Raise the affected part if possible. Place a cold compress such as an ice pack (p.241) on the affected area for at least ten minutes to minimize the risk of swelling.

3 Monitor vital signs—level of response, breathing, and pulse (pp.52–53). Watch for signs of an allergic reaction, such as wheezing and/or reddened, swollen, itchy skin.

RECOGNITION
Depends on the species, but generally:
- Pain, redness, and swelling at site of sting
- Nausea and vomiting
- Headache

YOUR AIMS
- To relieve pain and swelling
- To arrange removal to the hospital if necessary

SEE ALSO Allergy p.222 | Anaphylactic shock p.223 | The unconscious casualty pp.54–87

SNAKE BITE

RECOGNITION

There may be:

- A pair of puncture marks—the bite may be painless
- Severe pain, redness, and swelling at the bite
- Nausea and vomiting
- Disturbed vision
- Increased salivation and sweating
- Labored breathing; it may stop altogether

YOUR AIMS

- To prevent venom from spreading
- To arrange urgent removal to the hospital

While a snake bite is usually not serious, it is safer to assume that a snake is venomous if a person has been bitten. A venomous bite is often painless. Depending on the snake, venom may cause local tissue destruction; it may block nerve impulses, causing breathing and the heart to stop; or, cause blood clotting (coagulation) and then internal bleeding.

There are four groups of venomous snakes in the US: rattlesnakes, copperheads, water moccasins, and coral snakes. Do not attempt to kill or capture the snake that bit the casualty. But, if possible, make a note of the snake's appearance to help doctors identify the correct antivenom. Take precautions to prevent other people from being bitten. The first aid principles for treating any kind of snake bite are the same.

WHAT TO DO

1 Help the casualty lie down, with head and shoulders raised. Reassure the casualty and advise her not to move the bitten limb to prevent venom from spreading. **Call 911 for emergency help.**

2 If you have been properly trained, consider wrapping a pressure bandage around the entire length of the limb that was bitten. The bandage should be comfortably snug but loose enough to allow a finger to be slipped under it.

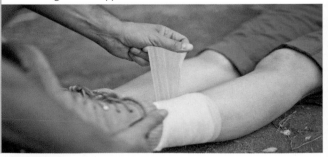

3 Whether or not it is wrapped, the bitten limb should be immobilized with a splint to prevent the casualty from bending it. Keep the limb below the level of the heart.

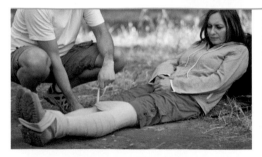

4 **Monitor and record** vital signs (pp.52–53) while waiting for emergency help. The casualty must remain still, and should be taken to the hospital as soon as possible.

STINGS FROM SEA CREATURES

Jellyfish, Portuguese man o' wars, sea anemones, and corals can all cause stings. Their venom is contained in stinging cells that stick to the casualty's skin. Most marine species found in temperate regions are not dangerous. However, some tropical marine creatures can cause severe poisoning. Death may result from paralysis of the chest muscles or, rarely, anaphylactic shock (p.223).

WHAT TO DO

1 Encourage the casualty to sit or lie down. **Wash the area** in copious quantities of vinegar to remove the stinging cells (nematocysts) or deactivate the venom.

2 To treat pain after venom has been deactivated, immerse the affected area in hot water.

3 Monitor vital signs—level of response, breathing, and pulse (pp.52–53). Watch for signs of an allergic reaction, such as wheezing.

SPECIAL CASE
JELLYFISH STING

Pour copious amounts of vinegar over the area of the injury to incapacitate the stinging cells. Help the casualty sit down. **Call 911 for emergency help.**

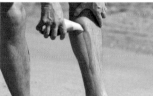

CAUTION

■ If the injury is extensive or there is a severe reaction, **call 911 for emergency help**. Monitor and record vital signs—level of response, breathing, and pulse (pp.52–53)—while waiting for help to arrive.

RECOGNITION

Depends on the species, but generally:

■ Pain, redness, and swelling at site of sting
■ Nausea and vomiting
■ Headache

YOUR AIMS

■ To relieve pain and discomfort
■ To seek medical help if necessary

MARINE PUNCTURE WOUND

Many marine creatures have spines that provide a mechanism against attack from predators but that can also cause painful wounds if stepped on. Sea urchins and weever fish have sharp spines that can become embedded in the sole of the foot. Wounds may become infected if the spines are not removed. Hot water breaks down fish venom.

CAUTION

■ Do not bandage the wound.
■ Do not scald the casualty.

YOUR AIM

■ To relieve pain and discomfort

WHAT TO DO

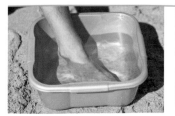

1 Help the casualty sit down. Immerse the injured part in water as hot as he can tolerate for about 30 minutes.

2 Take or send the casualty to the hospital so that the spines can be safely removed.

SEE ALSO Allergy p.222 | Anaphylactic shock **p.223** **207**

10

Many everyday conditions, such as fever and headache, need prompt treatment and respond well to first aid. However, a minor complaint can be the start of serious illness, so you should always be alert to this and seek medical advice if you are in doubt about the casualty's condition.

Other conditions such as heart attack, diabetes-related hypoglycemia (lower-than-normal blood sugar levels), severe allergic reaction (anaphylaxis), and meningitis are potentially life-threatening and require urgent medical attention.

Childbirth is a natural process and often takes many hours. So when a woman goes into labor unexpectedly, while it is important to call for emergency help, there is usually plenty of time to seek help and get her to the hospital. In the rare event of a baby arriving quickly, do not try to deliver the baby—the birth will happen naturally without intervention.

Miscarriage, however, is a potentially serious problem due to the risk of severe bleeding. A woman who is miscarrying needs urgent medical help.

AIMS AND OBJECTIVES

- To assess the casualty's condition quietly and calmly
- To comfort and reassure the casualty
- To **call 911 for emergency help** if you suspect a serious illness

MEDICAL
CONDITIONS

ANGINA

CAUTION

- If the casualty becomes unconscious and is not breathing normally, begin CPR with chest compressions (pp.54–87).

The **term angina** means literally a constriction of the chest. Angina occurs when coronary arteries that supply the heart muscle with blood become narrowed and cannot carry sufficient blood to meet increased demands during exertion or excitement. An attack forces the casualty to rest; the pain should ease soon afterward.

RECOGNITION

- Vicelike central chest pain, which may spread to the jaw and down one or both arms
- Pain easing with rest
- Shortness of breath
- Fatigue, which is often sudden and extreme
- Feeling of anxiety

YOUR AIMS

- To ease strain on the heart by ensuring that the casualty rests
- To help the casualty with any medication
- To obtain medical help if necessary

WHAT TO DO

1 **Help the casualty stop** what he is doing and sit down. Make sure that he is comfortable and reassure him; this should help the pain to ease.

2 **If the casualty has angina medication,** such as tablets or a pump-action or aerosol spray, let him administer it himself. If necessary, help him take it.

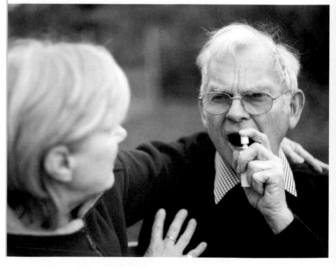

3 **If the pain is not relieved** five minutes after taking the angina medication, advise him to take a second dose.

4 **Encourage the casualty to rest,** and keep any bystanders away.

5 **If the casualty is still in pain** five minutes after the second dose, or it returns, suspect a heart attack (opposite). **Call 911 for emergency help.**

6 **If the pain subsides after rest** and/or medication, the casualty will usually be able to resume what he was doing. If he is concerned, tell him to seek medical advice.

HEART ATTACK

A heart attack is most commonly caused by a sudden obstruction of the blood supply to part of the heart muscle—for example, because of a clot in a coronary artery (coronary thrombosis). It can also be called a myocardial infarction. The main risk is that the heart will stop beating.

The effects of a heart attack depend largely on how much of the heart muscle is affected; many casualities recover completely. Aspirin can be used to try to limit the extent of damage to the heart muscle.

Coronary thrombosis
Coronary arteries supply blood to the heart muscle. When an artery is blocked, for example by a blood clot, the muscle beyond the blockage is deprived of oxygen and other nutrients carried by the blood, and begins to die.

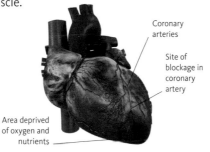

Coronary arteries

Site of blockage in coronary artery

Area deprived of oxygen and nutrients

RECOGNITION

- Persistent, vicelike central chest pain, which may spread to the jaw and down one or both arms. Unlike angina (opposite), the pain does not ease when the casualty rests.
- Breathlessness
- Discomfort occurring high in the abdomen, which may feel similar to severe indigestion
- Collapse, often without any warning
- Sudden faintness or dizziness
- Casualty feels a sense of impending doom
- "Ashen" skin and blueness at the lips
- A rapid, weak, or irregular pulse
- Profuse sweating
- Extreme gasping for air ("air hunger")

YOUR AIMS

- To ease the strain on the casualty's heart by ensuring that he rests
- To call for urgent medical help without delay

WHAT TO DO

1 Call **911** for emergency help. Tell the dispatcher that you suspect a heart attack. If the casualty asks you to do so, call his own doctor too.

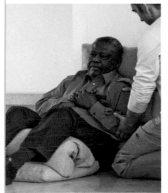

3 **Assist the casualty** to take up to one full-dose adult aspirin tablet (325 mg) or four baby aspirin (81 mg each). Advise him to chew it slowly.

4 **If the casualty has angina medication,** such as tablets or a pump-action or aerosol spray, let him administer it; help him if necessary. Encourage him to rest.

5 **Monitor and record vital signs**—level of response, breathing, and pulse (pp.52–53) —while waiting for help. Stay calm to avoid undue stress.

2 **Make the casualty as comfortable as possible** to ease the strain on his heart. A half-sitting position, with his head and shoulders supported and his knees bent, is often best. Place cushions behind him and under his knees.

STROKE

RECOGNITION

- Facial weakness—the casualty is unable to smile evenly and the mouth or eye may be droopy
- Arm weakness—the casualty is only able to raise one arm
- Speech problems—the casualty is unable to speak clearly

There may also be:

- Sudden weakness or numbness of the face, arm, or leg on one or both sides of the body
- Sudden loss or blurring of vision in one or both eyes
- Sudden difficulty with speech or understanding the spoken word
- Sudden confusion
- Sudden severe headache with no apparent cause
- Dizziness, unsteadiness, or sudden fall

YOUR AIMS

- To arrange urgent admission to the hospital
- To reassure and comfort the casualty

A stroke or brain attack is a medical emergency that occurs when the blood supply to the brain is disrupted. Strokes are the third most common cause of death in the US and many people live with long-term disability as a result of a stroke. This condition is more common later in life and is associated with disorders of the circulatory system, such as high blood pressure.

The majority of strokes are caused by a clot in a blood vessel that blocks the flow of blood to the brain. However, some strokes are the result of a ruptured blood vessel that causes bleeding into the brain. If a stroke is due to a blood clot, it may be possible to give drugs to limit the extent of damage to the brain and improve recovery. The earlier the casualty receives care in the hospital, the better.

Use the FAST (Face-Arm-Speech-Time) guide if you suspect a casualty has had a stroke:

F – Facial weakness—the casualty is unable to smile evenly and the mouth or eye may be droopy

A – Arm weakness—the casualty is only able to raise one of his arms

S – Speech problems—the casualty is unable to speak clearly or may not understand the spoken word

T – Time to **call 911 for emergency help** if you suspect that the casualty has had a stroke.

TRANSIENT ISCHEMIC ATTACK (TIA)

A transient ischemic attack, or TIA, is sometimes called a mini-stroke. It is similar to a full stroke, but the symptoms may last only a few minutes, will improve, and eventually disappear. If you suspect a TIA, it is important to seek medical advice to confirm the casualty's condition. If there is any doubt, assume that it is a stroke.

Causes of a stroke

Any disruption to the flow of blood to the brain starves the affected part of the brain of oxygen and nutrients. This can cause temporary or permanent loss of function in that area of the brain. A stroke can result from a blood clot that blocks an artery supplying blood to the brain (right), or from a burst blood vessel that causes bleeding which presses on the brain (far right).

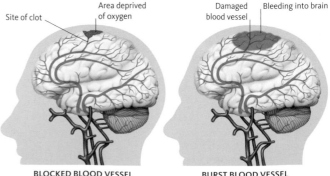

Site of clot — Area deprived of oxygen   Damaged blood vessel — Bleeding into brain

BLOCKED BLOOD VESSEL   **BURST BLOOD VESSEL**

WHAT TO DO

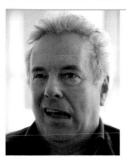

1 Look at the casualty's face. Ask him to smile; if he has had a stroke he may only be able to smile on one side—the other side of his mouth may droop.

2 Ask the casualty to raise both his arms; if he has had a stroke, he may be able to lift only one arm.

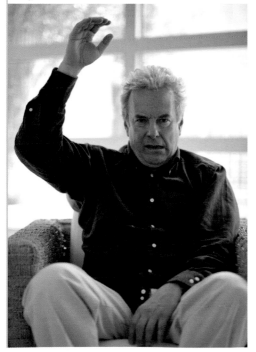

3 Find out whether the person can speak clearly and understand what you say. When you ask a question, does he respond appropriately to you?

4 Call 911 for emergency help. Tell the dispatcher that you have used the FAST guide and you suspect a stroke.

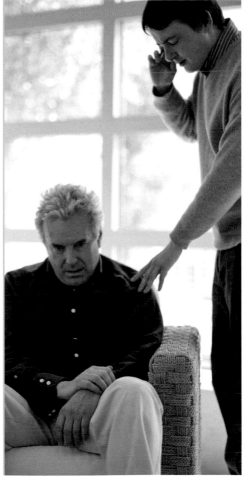

5 Keep the casualty comfortable and supported. If the casualty is conscious, you can help him lie down. Reassure him that help is on the way.

6 Regularly monitor and record vital signs—level of response, breathing, and pulse (pp.52–53)—while waiting for help to arrive. Do not give the casualty anything to eat or drink because it may be difficult for him to swallow.

DIABETES MELLITUS

This is a long-term (chronic) condition in which the body fails to produce sufficient insulin. Insulin is a chemical produced by the pancreas (a gland that lies behind the stomach), which regulates the blood sugar (glucose) level in the body. Diabetes can result in higher than normal blood sugar (hyperglycemia) or lower than normal blood sugar (hypoglycemia). If a person with diabetes is unwell, giving him sugar will rapidly correct hypoglycemia and is unlikely to do harm in cases of hyperglycemia.

TYPES OF DIABETES

There are two types: Type 1, or insulin-dependent diabetes, and Type 2, also known as non-insulin-dpendent diabetes.

In Type 1 diabetes, the body produces little or no insulin. People with Type 1 diabetes need regular insulin injections throughout their lives. Type 1 diabetes is sometimes referred to as juvenile diabetes or early-onset diabetes because it usually develops in childhood or the teenage years. Insulin can be administered using an insulin syringe, an injection pen, or a special pump. The pump is a small device about the size of a pack of cards, strapped to the person's body. The insulin is administered via a piece of tubing that leads from the pump to a needle just under the skin.

In Type 2 diabetes, the body does not make enough insulin or cannot use it properly. This type is usually linked with obesity, and is also known as maturity-onset diabetes because it is more common in people over the age of 40. The risk of developing this type is increased if it runs in your family. Type 2 diabetes can sometimes be controlled with diet, weight loss, and regular exercise. However, oral medication and, in some cases, insulin injections may be needed.

HYPERGLYCEMIA

High blood sugar (hyperglycemia) may develop slowly over a period of hours or days. If it is not treated, hyperglycemia will result in unconsciousness (diabetic coma) and therefore requires urgent treatment in the hospital. Those who suffer from hyperglycemia may wear warning bracelets, cards, or medallions alerting a first aider to the condition.

CAUTION

- If the casualty loses consciousness and is not breathing (or just gasping), begin CPR with chest compressions (pp.54–87).

RECOGNITION

- Warm, dry skin
- Rapid pulse and breathing
- Fruity sweet breath and excessive thirst
- Drowsiness, leading to unconsciousness if untreated

YOUR AIM

- To arrange urgent removal to the hospital.

WHAT TO DO

1 **Call 911 for emergency help;** tell dispatcher that you suspect hyperglycemia.

2 **Monitor and record** vital signs—level of response, breathing, and pulse (pp.52–53)—while waiting for help to arrive.

HYPOGLYCEMIA

This condition occurs when the blood sugar level falls below normal. It is characterized by a rapidly deteriorating level of response. Hypoglycemia develops if the insulin–sugar balance is incorrect; for example, when a person with diabetes misses a meal or does too much exercise. It is common in a person with newly diagnosed diabetes while he is learning to balance sugar levels. More rarely, hypoglycemia may develop following an epileptic seizure (pp.216–17) or after an episode of binge drinking.

People with diabetes may carry their own blood-testing kits to check their blood sugar levels, as well as their insulin medication, so they are well prepared for emergencies; for example, many carry sugar, candy, or a tube of glucose gel.

If the hypoglycemic attack is at an advanced stage, consciousness may be impaired and you must seek emergency help.

CAUTION

- If consciousness is impaired, do not give the casualty anything to eat or drink.
- If the person loses consciousness and is not breathing (or just gasping), begin CPR with chest compressions (pp.54–87).

RECOGNITION

There may be:

- A history of diabetes—the casualty himself may recognize the onset of a hypoglycemic attack
- Weakness, faintness, or hunger
- Confusion and irrational behavior
- Sweating with cold, clammy skin
- Rapid pulse
- Palpitations and muscle tremors
- Deteriorating level of response
- Medical warning bracelet or necklace, and glucose gel or tablets
- Medication such as an insulin pen or tablets, and a glucose testing kit

YOUR AIMS

- To raise the sugar content of the blood as quickly as possible
- To obtain appropriate medical help

WHAT TO DO

1 **Help the casualty sit down.** If he has his own glucose gel or tablets, help him take it. If not, give him the equivalent of 10 g of glucose—for example, an 8 oz glass of nondiet carbonated beverage or fruit juice, two teaspoons of sugar (or two lumps of sugar), or sugary candy such as hard candies.

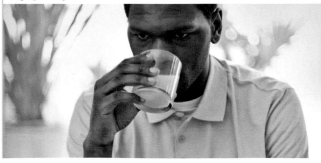

2 **If the casualty responds quickly,** give him more food or drink and let him rest until he feels better. Help him find his glucose testing kit so that he can check his glucose level. Monitor him until he is completely recovered.

3 **If the casualty's condition does not improve,** look for other possible causes. **Call 911 for emergency help** and monitor and record vital signs—level of response, breathing, and pulse (pp.52–53)—while waiting for help to arrive.

SEE ALSO Alcohol poisoning p.202 | Head injury pp.144–45 | The unconscious casualty pp.54–87

SEIZURES IN ADULTS

A seizure—also called a convulsion—consists of involuntary contractions of many of the muscles in the body. The condition is due to a disturbance in the electrical activity of the brain. Seizures usually result in loss or impairment of consciousness. The most common cause is epilepsy. Other causes include head injury, some brain-damaging diseases, shortage of oxygen or glucose in the brain, and the intake of certain poisons, including alcohol or drugs.

Epileptic seizures result from recurrent, major disturbances of brain activity. These seizures can be sudden and dramatic. Just before a seizure, a casualty may have a brief warning period (aura) with, for example, a strange feeling or a particular smell or taste.

No matter what the cause of the seizure, care must always include maintaining an open, clear airway and a monitoring of the casualty's vital signs—level of response, breathing, and pulse. You will also need to protect the casualty from further harm during a seizure and arrange appropriate aftercare once he has recovered.

SPECIAL CASE ABSENCE SEIZURES

Some people experience a mild form of epilepsy known as absence seizures, during which they appear distant and unaware of their surroundings. These seizures tend to affect children more than adults, and a more severe seizure with convulsions may follow. A casualty may suddenly "switch off" and stare blankly ahaed. You may notice slight or localized twitching or jerking of the lips, eyelids, head, or limbs and/ or odd "automatic" movements, such as lip-smacking or making noises. If a casualty has an absence seizure:

- Help him sit down in a quiet place
- Remove any potentially dangerous items such as hot drinks and sharp objects
- Talk to him in a calm and reassuring way and stay with him until he has fully recovered
- Advise him to seek medical advice if he is unaware of his condition or does not fully recover.

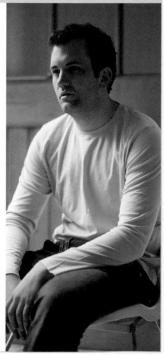

WHAT TO DO

1 Make space around the casualty, and ask bystanders to move away. Remove potentially dangerous items, such as hot drinks and sharp objects. Note the time that the seizure started.

2 Protect the casualty's head from objects nearby; place soft padding such as rolled towels underneath or around his neck if possible. Loosen tight clothing around his neck if necessary.

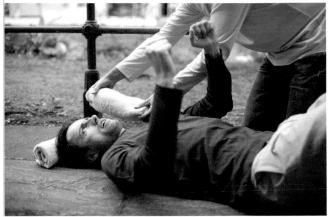

3 When the convulsive movements have ceased, open the casualty's airway and check breathing. If he is breathing, place him in the recovery position.

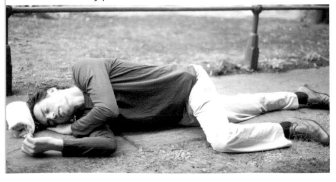

4 Monitor and record his vital signs—level of response, breathing, and pulse (pp.52–53)—until he recovers. Make a note of how long the seizure lasted.

RECOGNITION

In epilepsy, the following sequence is common:

- Sudden loss of consciousness
- Casualty becomes rigid and arches his back
- Breathing may be noisy and become difficult—the lips may show a gray-blue tinge (cyanosis)
- Convulsive movements begin
- Saliva may appear at the mouth and may be bloodstained if the lips or tongue have been bitten
- Possible loss of bladder or bowel control
- Muscles relax and breathing becomes normal; the casualty recovers consciousness, usually within a few minutes. He may feel dazed, or act strangely. He may be unaware of his actions
- After a seizure, the casualty may feel tired and fall into a deep sleep

YOUR AIMS

- To protect the casualty from injury during the seizure
- To care for the casualty when consciousness is regained and arrange removal to the hospital if necessary

SEE ALSO Head injury **pp.144–45** | The unconscious casualty **pp.54–87**

SEIZURES IN CHILDREN

RECOGNITION

- Vigorous shaking, with clenched fists and an arched back.

There may also be:

- Obvious signs of fever: hot, flushed skin and perhaps sweating
- Twitching of the face and squinting, fixed or upturned eyes
- Breath-holding, with red, "puffy" face and neck and drooling
- Possible vomiting
- Loss of bowel or bladder control
- Loss of or impaired consciousness

YOUR AIMS

- To protect the child from injury during the seizure
- To cool the child
- To reassure the parents
- To arrange removal to the hospital

In young children, seizures—sometimes called convulsions—are most often the result of a raised body temperature associated with a throat or ear infection or other infections. This type of seizure, also known as a febrile seizure, occurs because the electrical systems in the brain are not mature enough to deal with the body's high temperature.

Although seizures can be alarming, they are rarely dangerous if properly dealt with. However, you should always seek medical advice for the child to rule out any serious underlying condition.

WHAT TO DO

1 **Place pillows or soft padding** around the child so that even violent movement will not result in injury. Do not restrain the child in any way.

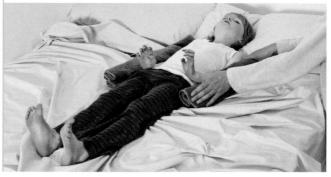

2 **If the child's seizure** was caused by a fever, cool him by removing any bedding and clothes, for example T-shirt or pajama top; you may have to wait until the seizure stops. Ensure a good supply of fresh air (but do not overcool the child).

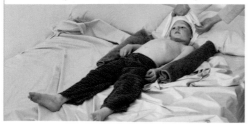

3 **Once the seizures** have stopped, maintain an open airway by placing the casualty in the recovery position. **Call 911 for emergency help.**

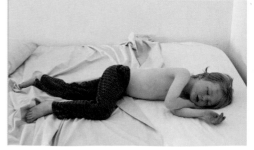

4 **Reassure the child** as well as the parents or caregiver. Monitor and record vital signs—level of response, breathing, and pulse (pp.52–53)—until emergency help arrives.

FEVER

The normal body temperature varies, but it is approximately 98.6°F (37°C). Fever is generally defined as a temperature over 100.4°F (38°C). It is usually caused by a bacterial or viral infection, and may be associated with earache, sore throat, measles, chickenpox, meningitis (p.220) or local infection, such as an abscess. The infection may have been acquired during overseas travel.

In young children, fever can be a symptom of or a precursor to serious illnesses. See list at right, and if you are in any doubt about a casualty's condition, seek medical advice.

CAUTION

- If you are concerned about the casualty's condition, seek medical advice.
- Do not over- or under-dress a child with fever; do not sponge a child to cool her because there is a risk of overcooling.
- Do not give aspirin to any person under 16 years of age.

WHAT TO DO

1 Keep casualty cool and comfortable—preferably in bed with a light covering.

2 Give her plenty of cool drinks to replace body fluids lost through sweating.

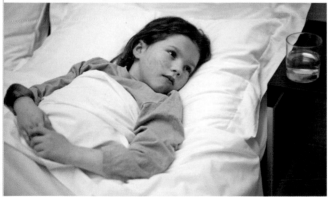

3 If the child appears distressed or ill, she may have the recommended dose of acetaminophen syrup (not aspirin). An adult may take the recommended dose of acetaminophen or ibuprofen, or his own pain relievers.

4 Monitor and record a casualty's vital signs—level of response, breathing, pulse, and temperature (pp.52–53)—until she recovers.

RECOGNITION

- Raised body temperature above 100.4°F (38°C)
- Pallor; casualty may feel cold with goose pimples, shivering, and chattering teeth

Later:
- Hot, flushed skin and sweating
- Headache
- Generalized aches and pains

YOUR AIMS

- To bring down the fever

To obtain medical aid if necessary, for:

- An infant less than 3 months of age with a rectal temperature of 100.4°F (38°C) or higher
- A child 3 months – 3 years old with a rectal temperature of 100.4°F (38°C) or higher for more than three days or who appears ill or fussy
- A child 3 months – 3 years old with a rectal temperature of 102°F (38.9°C) or higher
- A child of any age with a temperature of 104°F (40°C) or higher
- A child of any age who has a febrile seizure
- A child of any age who has a chronic medical problem
- An infant or child of any age who has a fever as well as a new skin rash

SEE ALSO | Meningitis **p.220** | Seizures in children **opposite**

MENINGITIS

RECOGNITION

The symptoms and signs are usually not all present at the same time. They include:

- Flulike illness with a high temperature
- Cold hands and feet
- Joint and limb pain
- Mottled or very pale skin.

As the infection develops:

- Severe headache
- Neck stiffness (the casualty will not be able to touch her chest with her chin)
- Vomiting
- Eyes become very sensitive to any light—daylight, electric light, or even the television
- Drowsiness
- In infants, there may also be high-pitched moaning or a whimpering cry, floppiness, and a tense or bulging fontanelle (soft part of the skull)

Later:

- A distinctive rash of red or purple spots that do not fade when pressed

YOUR AIM

- To obtain urgent medical help

This is a condition in which the linings that surround the brain and the spinal cord become inflamed. It can be caused by bacteria or a virus and can affect any age group.

Meningitis may be a very serious illness and the casualty may deteriorate very quickly. If you suspect meningitis, you must seek urgent medical assistance because prompt treatment in the hospital is vital. For this reason it is important that you can recognize the symptoms of meningitis, which may include a high temperature, headache, and a distinctive rash. With early diagnosis and treatment, full recovery is possible.

WHAT TO DO

1 Seek urgent medical advice if you notice any of the signs of meningitis; for example, shielding eyes from the light. Do not wait for all the symptoms and signs to appear because they may not all develop. Treat the fever p.219.

2 Check the casualty for signs of a rash. On dark skin, check on lighter parts of the body; for example, the inner eyelids or fingertips. If you see any signs, **call 911 for emergency help.**

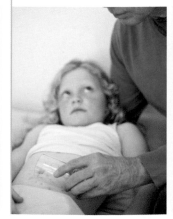

3 While waiting for help to arrive, reassure the casualty and keep her cool. Monitor and record vital signs—level of response, breathing, and pulse (pp.52–53).

IMPORTANT MENINGITIS RASH

Accompanying the later stage of meningitis is a distinctive red or purple rash that does not fade if you press it. If you press the side of a glass firmly against most rashes they will fade; if a rash does not fade, **call 911 for emergency** help immediately.

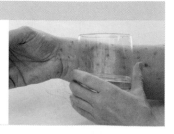

FAINTING

Fainting is a brief loss of consciousness caused by a temporary reduction of the blood flow to the brain. It may be a reaction to pain, exhaustion, lack of food, or emotional stress. It is also common after long periods of physical inactivity, such as standing or sitting still, especially in a warm atmosphere. This inactivity causes blood to pool in the legs, reducing the amount of blood reaching the brain.

When a person faints, the pulse rate becomes very slow. However, the rate soon picks up and returns to normal. A casualty who has fainted usually makes a rapid and complete recovery. Do not advise a person who feels faint to sit on a chair with his head between his knees because if he faints he may fall and injure himself. If the casualty is a woman in the late stages of pregnancy, help her lie down so that she is leaning toward her left side to prevent the pregnant uterus from restricting blood flow back to her heart.

CAUTION

- If the casualty does not regain consciousness quickly and is not breathing normally, begin CPR with compressions (pp.54–87).

RECOGNITION

- Brief loss of consciousness that causes the casualty to fall to the ground
- A slow pulse
- Pale, cold skin and sweating

YOUR AIMS

- To improve blood flow to the brain
- To reassure the casualty and make him comfortable

WHAT TO DO

1 When a casualty feels **faint,** advise him to lie down. Kneel down, raise his legs, supporting his ankles on your shoulders to improve blood flow to the brain. Watch his face for signs of recovery.

2 Make sure that the casualty has plenty of fresh air; ask someone to open a window if you are indoors. In addition, ask any bystanders to stand clear. He may be more comfortable if his knees are bent.

3 As the casualty recovers, reassure him and help him sit up gradually. If he starts to feel faint again, advise him to lie down once again, and raise and support his legs until he recovers fully.

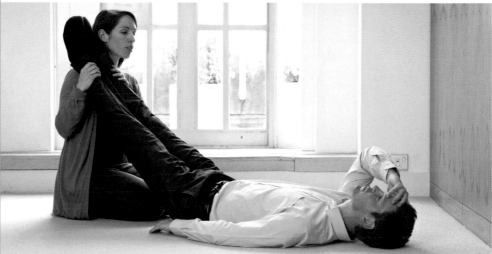

ALLERGY

RECOGNITION

Features of mild allergy vary depending on the trigger and the person. There may be:

- Red, itchy rash or raised areas of skin (hives)
- Red, itchy eyes
- Wheezing and/or difficulty breathing
- Swelling of hands, feet, and/or face
- Abdominal pain, vomiting, and diarrhea

YOUR AIMS

- To assess the severity of the allergic reaction
- To seek medical advice if necessary

An allergy is an abnormal reaction of the body's defense system (immune response) to a normally harmless "trigger" substance (or allergen). An allergy can present itself as a mild itching, swelling, wheezing, or digestive condition, or can progress to full-blown anaphylaxis, or anaphylactic shock (opposite), which can occur within seconds or minutes of exposure to an offending allergen.

Common allergy triggers include pollen, dust, nuts, shellfish, eggs, wasp and bee stings, latex, and certain medications. Skin changes can be subtle, absent, or variable in some cases.

WHAT TO DO

1 Assess the casualty's signs and symptoms. Ask if she has any known allergy.

2 **Remove the trigger** if possible, or move the casualty from the trigger.

3 **Treat any symptoms.** Allow the casualty to take her own medication for a known allergy.

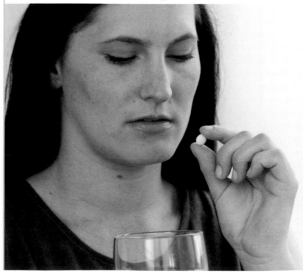

4 **If you are at all concerned** about the casualty's condition, seek medical advice.

ANAPHYLACTIC SHOCK

This is a severe allergic reaction affecting the whole body. It may develop within seconds or minutes of contact with a trigger and is potentially fatal. In an anaphylactic reaction, chemicals are released into the blood that widen (dilate) blood vessels. This causes blood pressure to fall and air passages to narrow (constrict), resulting in breathing difficulties. In addition, the tongue and throat can swell, obstructing the airway. The amount of oxygen reaching the vital organs can be severely reduced, causing hypoxia (p.92). Common triggers include: nuts, shellfish, eggs, wasp and bee stings, latex, and certain medications.

A casualty with anaphylactic shock needs emergency treatment with an injection of epinephrine.

CAUTION

- If a pregnant casualty needs to lie down, lean her toward her left side to prevent the pregnant uterus from restricting blood flow back to the heart.
- If the casualty loses consciousness and is not breathing normally, begin CPR with chest compressions (pp.54–87).

WHAT TO DO

1 **Call 911 for emergency help.** Tell the dispatcher that you suspect anaphylaxis.

2 **If the casualty** has an auto-injector of epinephrine, help her use it. If she is unable to take the medication, administer it to her yourself. Pull off the safety cap and, holding the injector with your fist, push the tip firmly against the casualty's thigh until it clicks, releasing the medication (it can be delivered through clothing). Hold for ten seconds, remove the autoinjector, then massage the injection site for ten seconds.

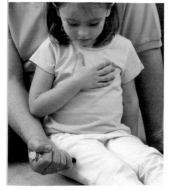

3 **Help the casualty sit up** in the position that best relieves any breathing difficulty. If she becomes pale with a weak pulse, help her lie down with legs raised and treat for shock (pp.112–113).

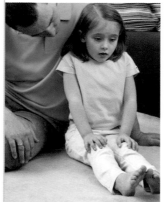

4 **Monitor and record** vital signs—level of response, breathing, and pulse (pp.52–53)—while waiting for help to arrive. Repeated doses of epinephrine can be given at five-minute intervals if there is no improvement or the symptoms return.

RECOGNITION

Features of allergy (opposite) may be present:

- Red, itchy rash or raised areas of skin (hives)
- Red itchy, watery eyes
- Swelling of hands, feet, and/or face
- Abdominal pain, vomiting, and diarrhea

There may also be:

- Difficulty breathing, ranging from a tight chest to severe difficulty, causing the casualty to wheeze and gasp for air
- Pale or flushed skin
- Visible swelling of tongue and throat with puffiness around the eyes
- Feeling of terror
- Confusion and agitation
- Signs of shock, leading to collapse and loss of consciousness

YOUR AIMS

- To ease breathing
- To treat shock
- To arrange urgent removal to the hospital

HEADACHE

YOUR AIMS

- To relieve the pain
- To obtain medical advice if necessary

A headache may accompany any illness, particularly a feverish ailment such as flu. It may develop for no reason, but can often be traced to fatigue, tension, stress, or undue heat or cold. Mild "poisoning" caused by a stuffy or fume-filled atmosphere, or by excess alcohol or any other drug, can also induce a headache. However, a headache may also be the most prominent symptom of meningitis or a stroke.

WHAT TO DO

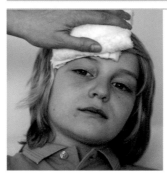

1 **Help the casualty** sit or lie down in a quiet place. Give him a cold compress to hold against his head (p.241).

2 **An adult may take** the recommended dose of acetaminophen tablets or his own pain relievers. A child may have the recommended dose of acetaminophen syrup (not aspirin).

MIGRAINE

RECOGNITION

- Before the attack there may be disturbance of vision in the form of flickering lights or an aura
- Intense throbbing headache, which is sometimes on just one side of the head
- Abdominal pain, nausea, and vomiting
- Inability to tolerate bright light or loud noise

YOUR AIMS

- To relieve the pain
- To obtain medical aid if necessary

Migraine attacks are severe, "sickening" headaches and can be triggered by a variety of causes, such as allergy, stress, or fatigue. Other triggers include lack of sleep, missed meals, alcohol, and some foods—for example, cheese or chocolate. Migraine sufferers usually know how to recognize and deal with attacks and may carry their own medication.

WHAT TO DO

1 **Help the casualty take** any medication that he may have for migraine attacks.

2 **Advise the casualty to lie** down or sleep for a few hours in a quiet, dark room. Provide him with some towels and a container in case he vomits.

3 **If this is the first attack,** advise the casualty to seek medical advice.

SORE THROAT

The most common sore throat is a "raw" feeling caused by inflammation, which is often the first sign of a cough or cold. Tonsillitis occurs when the tonsils at the back of the throat are infected. The tonsils become red and swollen and white spots of pus may be seen. Swallowing may be difficult and the glands at the angle of the jaw may be enlarged and sore.

CAUTION
- Do not give aspirin to anyone under 16 years of age.
- If you suspect tonsillitis, tell the casualty to seek medical advice.

WHAT TO DO

1 Give the casualty plenty of cold fluids to help ease the pain and keep the throat from becoming dry.

2 An adult may take the recommended dose of acetaminophen tablets or his own pain relievers. A child may have acetaminophen syrup.

YOUR AIMS
- To relieve the pain
- To obtain medical advice if necessary

EARACHE AND TOOTHACHE

Earache can result from inflammation of the outer, middle, or inner ear, often caused by an infection associated with a cold, tonsillitis, or flu. It can also be caused by a boil, an object stuck in the ear canal, or transmitted pain from a tooth abscess. There may also be temporary hearing loss. Earache often occurs when flying as a result of the changes in air pressure during ascent and descent. Infection can cause pus to collect in the middle ear; the eardrum may rupture, allowing the pus to drain, which temporarily eases the pain.

Toothache can develop when pulp inside a tooth becomes inflamed due to dental decay. If untreated, the pulp becomes infected, leading to an abscess, which causes a throbbing pain. Infection may cause swelling around the tooth or jaw.

CAUTION
- Do not give aspirin to anyone under 16 years of age.
- If there is a discharge from an ear, fever, or hearing loss, obtain medical help.

YOUR AIMS
- To relieve the pain
- To obtain medical or dental advice if necessary

WHAT TO DO

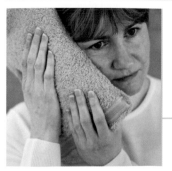

1 An adult may take the recommended dose of acetaminophen or ibuprofen tablets or her own pain relievers. A child may have the recommended dose of acetaminophen syrup.

2 Give her a source of heat, such as a hot water bottle wrapped in a towel, to hold against the affected side of her face.

3 For toothache, you can apply benzocaine, in many tooth pain products, to the painful tooth.

4 Advise a casualty to seek medical advice if you are concerned, particularly if the casualty is a child. If a casualty has toothache, advise her to see her dentist.

SEE ALSO Foreign object in the ear **p.197**

ABDOMINAL PAIN

YOUR AIMS

- To relieve pain and discomfort
- To obtain medical help if necessary

Pain in the abdomen often has a relatively minor cause, such as food poisoning. The pain of a stitch usually occurs during exercise and is sharp. Distension (widening) or obstruction of the intestine causes colic—pain that comes and goes in waves—which often makes the casualty double up in agony and may be accompanied by vomiting.

Occasionally abdominal pain is a sign of a serious disorder affecting the organs and other structures in the abdomen. If the appendix bursts, or the intestine is damaged, the contents of the intestine can leak into the abdominal cavity, causing inflammation of the cavity lining. This life-threatening condition, called peritonitis, causes intense pain, which is made worse by movement or pressure on the abdomen, and will lead to shock (pp.112–13).

An inflamed appendix (appendicitis) is especially common in children. Symptoms include pain (often starting in the center of the abdomen and moving to the lower right-hand side), loss of appetite, nausea, vomiting, bad breath, and fever. If the appendix bursts, peritonitis will develop. The treatment is urgent surgical removal of the appendix.

WHAT TO DO

1 Reassure the casualty and make her comfortable. Prop her up if she finds breathing difficult. Give her a container to use if she is vomiting.

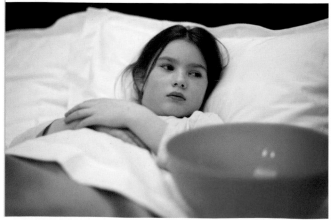

2 Give the casualty a hot-water bottle wrapped in a towel to hold against her abdomen. If in doubt about her condition, seek medical advice.

SPECIAL CASE STITCH

This common condition is a form of cramp, usually associated with exercise, which occurs in the trunk or the sides of the chest. The most likely cause is a buildup in the muscles of chemical waste products, such as lactic acid, during physical exertion. Help the casualty sit down and reassure him. The pain will usually ease quickly. If the pain does not disappear within a few minutes, or if you are concerned about the casualty's condition, seek medical advice.

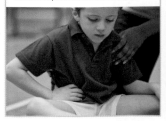

VOMITING AND DIARRHEA

These problems are usually due to irritation of the digestive system. Diarrhea and vomiting can be caused by a number of different organisms, including viruses, bacteria, and parasites. They usually result from consuming contaminated food or water, but infection can be passed from person to person. Good hygiene helps prevent infectious diarrhea.

Vomiting and diarrhea may occur either separately or together. Both conditions can cause the body to lose vital fluids and salts, resulting in dehydration. When they occur together, the risk of dehydration is increased and can be serious, especially in infants, young children, and elderly people.

The aim of treatment is to prevent dehydration by giving frequent sips of water or unsweetened fruit juice, even if the casualty is vomiting. Dehydration products, whether added to water or sold in liquid form, provide the correct balance of water and salt to replace those lost through the vomiting and diarrhea and can be purchased at a pharmacy.

CAUTION

- Do not give antidiarrhea medicines.
- If you are concerned about a casualty's condition, especially if the vomiting or diarrhea is persistent, or the casualty is a young child or an older person, seek medical advice.

RECOGNITION

There may be:
- Nausea
- Vomiting and later diarrhea
- Stomach pains
- Fever

YOUR AIMS

- To reassure the casualty
- To restore lost fluids and salts

WHAT TO DO

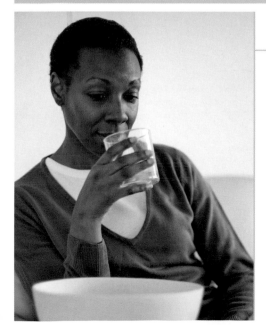

1 **Reassure the casualty** if she is vomiting and give her a warm damp cloth to wipe her face.

2 **Help her sit down** and when the vomiting stops give her water or unsweetened fruit juice to sip slowly and often.

3 **When the casualty is hungry** again, advise her to eat easily digested foods such as pasta, bread, or potatoes for the first 24 hours.

4 If the vomiting and/or diarrhea are severe, or the casualty develops chest pain, difficulty breathing, or severe abdominal pain, take or arrange to send her to the hospital. If the casualty becomes lightheaded or dizzy, treat for fainting (p.221).

SEE ALSO Drug poisoning **p.201** | Swallowed poisons **p.200**

CHILDBIRTH

Childbirth is a natural and often lengthy process that normally occurs at about the 40th week of pregnancy. There is usually plenty of time to get a woman to the hospital, or get help to her, before the baby arrives. Most pregnant women are aware of what happens during childbirth, but a woman who goes into labor unexpectedly or early may be very anxious. You will need to reassure her and make her comfortable. Miscarriage, however, is potentially serious because there is a risk of severe bleeding. A woman who is miscarrying needs urgent medical help (p.128).

There are three distinct stages to childbirth. In the first stage, the baby gets into position for the birth. The baby is born in the second stage, and in the third stage, the afterbirth (placenta and umbilical cord) is delivered.

Uterus contracts to push baby down | Baby's head presses against cervix

Birth canal fully dilated | Baby emerges

Placenta detaches from wall of uterus | Umbilical cord

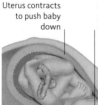
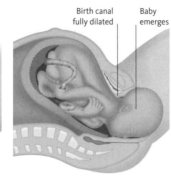

First stage
In this stage, a woman's body begins to experience contractions, which, together with the pressure of the baby's head, cause the cervix (neck of the uterus/womb) to open. The contractions become stronger and more frequent until the cervix is fully dilated (open)—about 4 in (10 cm)—and ready for the baby to be born. During this first stage, the mucous plug that protects the uterus from infection is expelled and the amniotic fluid surrounding the baby leaks out from the vagina. This stage can take several hours for a first baby but is normally shorter in any subsequent pregnancies.

Second stage
Once the cervix is fully dilated, the baby's head will press down on the mother's pelvic floor, triggering a strong urge to push. The birth canal (vagina) stretches as the baby travels through it. The baby's head normally emerges first, and the body is delivered soon afterward. This stage of labor normally lasts about an hour.

Third stage
About 10–30 minutes after the baby is born, the placenta (the organ that nourishes the unborn baby) and the umbilical cord will be expelled from the uterus. The uterus begins to contract again, pushing the placenta out, then it closes down the area where it was attached; this reduces the bleeding.

EMERGENCY CHILDBIRTH

In the rare event of a baby arriving quickly, you should not try to "deliver" the baby; the birth will happen naturally without intervention. Your role is to comfort and listen to the wishes of the mother and care for her and her baby.

CAUTION

- Do not give the mother anything to eat because there is a risk that she may vomit. If she is thirsty give her sips of water.
- Do not pull on the baby's head or shoulders during delivery.
- If the umbilical cord is wrapped around the baby's neck as he is born, check that it is loose, and then very carefully ease it over the baby's head to prevent strangulation.
- If a newborn baby does not cry, open the airway and check breathing (Unconscious infant pp. 80–83). Do not slap the baby.
- Do not pull or cut the umbilical cord, even when the placenta has been delivered.

WHAT TO DO

1 **Call 911 for emergency help.** Give the 911 dispatcher details of the stage the mother has reached, the length of each contraction and the intervals between them. Follow the instructions of the dispatcher.

2 **During the first stage,** help her sit or kneel on the floor in a comfortable position. Support her with cushions or let her move around. Stay calm, and encourage her to breathe deeply during her contractions.

3 **Massage her lower back gently** using the heel of your hand. She may find having her face and hands wiped soothing, or you can spray her face with cool water and give her ice cubes to suck.

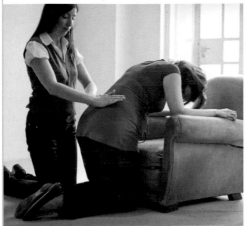

4 **When the second stage starts,** the mother will want to push. Make sure the surroundings are as clean as possible to reduce the risk of infection. The mother should remove any items of clothing that could interfere with the birth. Put clean sheets or towels under the woman; she may also want to be covered. Encourage her to stay as upright as possible.

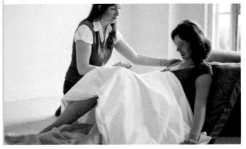

5 **As the baby is born,** handle him carefully—newborns are very slippery. Make sure he is breathing, wrap him in a clean cloth, towel, or blanket, and place him between his mother's legs so he is on the same level as the afterbirth.

6 **As the third stage begins,** reassure the mother. Support her as she delivers the afterbirth; do not cut the cord. Keep the placenta and the umbilical cord intact because the doctor or ambulance crew need to check that it is complete. If bleeding or pain is severe, treat for shock (pp.112–13). Help the mother lie down and raise her legs.

SEE ALSO Shock pp.112–13 | Vaginal bleeding p.128

11

This chapter outlines the techniques and procedures that underpin first aid, including moving a casualty and applying dressings and bandages. Usually, a first aider is not expected to move an injured person, but in some circumstances—such as when a casualty is in immediate danger—it may be necessary. The key principles for moving casualties are described here. Information is also given on making an assessment of the risks involved in moving a casualty or assisting a casualty to safety.

A guide to the equipment and materials commonly found in a first aid kit is given, with information on how and when to use them. Applying dressings and bandages effectively is an essential part of first aid: wounds usually require a dressing, and almost all injuries benefit from the support that bandages can give.

AIMS AND OBJECTIVES

- To assess the casualty's condition.
- To comfort and reassure the casualty.
- To maintain a casualty's privacy and dignity.
- To use a first aid technique relevant to the injury.
- To use dressings and bandages as needed.
- To apply good handling techniques if moving a casualty.
- To obtain appropriate help: **call 911 for emergency help** if you suspect serious injury or illness.

TECHNIQUES
AND EQUIPMENT

REMOVING CLOTHING

To make a thorough examination of a casualty, obtain an accurate diagnosis, or give treatment, you may have to remove some of his clothing. This should be done with the minimum of disturbance to the casualty and with his agreement if possible. Remove as little clothing as possible and do not damage clothing unless it is necessary. If you need to cut a garment, try to cut along the seams, keeping the clothing clear of the casualty's injury. Maintain the casualty's privacy and prevent exposure to cold. Stop if removing clothing increases the casualty's discomfort or pain.

REMOVING CLOTHING IN LOWER BODY INJURIES

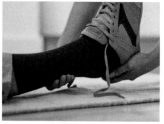

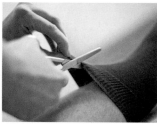

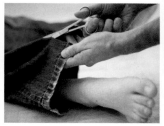

Shoes
Untie any laces, support the ankle, and carefully pull the shoe off by the heel. To remove long boots, you may need to cut them down the back seam.

Socks
Remove socks by pulling them off gently. If this is not possible, lift each sock away from the leg and cut the fabric with a pair of scissors.

Trousers
Gently pull up the pant leg to expose the calf and knee or pull down from the waist. If you need to cut clothing, lift it clear of the casualty's injury.

REMOVING CLOTHING IN UPPER BODY INJURIES

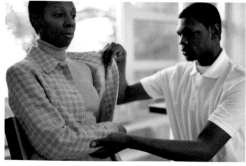

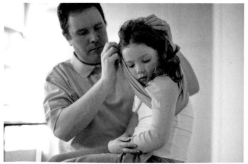

Jackets
Support the injured arm. Undo any fastenings on the jacket and gently pull the garment off the casualty's shoulders. Remove the arm on the uninjured side from its sleeve. Pull the garment around to the injured side of the body and ease it off the injured arm.

Sweaters and sweatshirts
With clothing that cannot be unfastened, begin by easing the arm on the uninjured side out of its sleeve. Next, roll up the garment and stretch it over the casualty's head. Finally, slip off the other sleeve of the garment, taking care not to disturb her arm on the injured side.

REMOVING HEADGEAR

Protective headgear, such as a a horseback rider's, bicyclist's, or motorcyclist's helmet, is best left on; it should be removed only if absolutely necessary, for example, if you cannot maintain an open airway. If the item does need to be removed, the casualty should do this herself if possible; otherwise, you and a helper should remove it. Support the head and neck at all times and keep the head aligned with the spine.

> **CAUTION**
>
> Do not remove a helmet unless absolutely necessary.

REMOVING AN OPEN-FACE OR RIDING HELMET

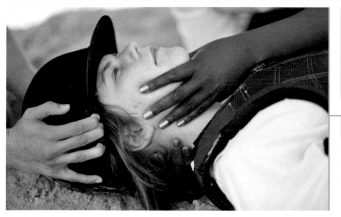

1 Undo or cut through the chinstrap. Support the casualty's head and neck, keeping them aligned with the spine. Hold the lower jaw with one hand and support the neck with the other hand.

2 Ask a helper to grip the sides of the helmet and pull them apart to take pressure off the head, then lift the helmet upward and backward.

REMOVING A FULL-FACE HELMET

1 Undo or cut the straps. Working from the base of the helmet, ease your fingers underneath the rim. Support the back of the neck with one hand and hold the lower jaw firmly. Ask a helper to hold the helmet with both hands.

2 Continue to support the casualty's neck and lower jaw. Ask your helper, working from above, to tilt the helmet backward (without moving the head) and gently lift the front of the helmet clear of the casualty's chin.

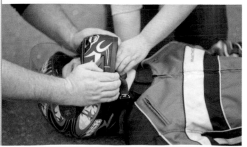

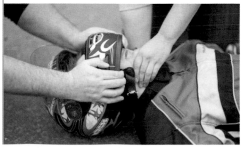

3 Maintain support on the head and neck. Ask your helper to tilt the helmet forward slightly so that it will pass over the base of the casualty's skull, and then to lift it straight off the casualty's head.

CASUALTY HANDLING

When giving first aid you should leave a casualty in the position in which you find him until medical help arrives. Only move him if he is in imminent danger, and even then only if it is safe for you to approach and you have the training and equipment to carry out the move. A casualty should be moved quickly if he is in imminent danger from:

- Drowning (p.100);
- Fire or he is in an area that is filling with smoke (pp.32–33);
- Explosion or gunfire;
- A collapsing building or other structure.

ASSESSING THE RISK OF MOVING A CASUALTY

If it is necessary to move a casualty, consider the following before you start.

- **Is the task necessary?** Usually, the casualty can be assessed and treated in the position in which you find him.
- **What are his injuries or conditions,** and will a move make them worse?
- **Can the casualty move himself?** Ask the casualty if he feels able to move.
- **The weight and size** of the casualty.
- **Can anyone help?** If so, are you and any helpers trained and physically fit?
- **Will you need protective equipment** to enter the area, and do you have it?
- **Is there any equipment available** to assist with moving the casualty and are you trained to use it?
- **Is there enough space** around the casualty to move him safely?
- **What sort of ground** will you be crossing?

ASSISTING A CASUALTY SAFELY

If you need to move a casualty, take the following steps to ensure safety.

- **Select a method relevant** to the situation, the casualty's condition, and the help and equipment that is available.
- **Use a team.** Appoint one person to coordinate the move and make sure that the team understands exactly what to do.
- **Plan your move** carefully and make sure that everyone is prepared.
- **Prepare any equipment** and make sure that the team and equipment are in position.
- **Use the correct technique** to avoid injuring the casualty, yourself, or any helpers.
- **Ensure the safety** and comfort of the casualty, yourself, and any helpers.
- **Always explain** to the casualty what is happening, and encourage him to cooperate as much as possible.
- **Position yourself** as close as possible to the casualty's body.
- **Adopt a stable base,** with your feet shoulder-width apart, so that you remain well balanced and maintain good posture at all times during the procedure.
- **Use the strongest muscles** in your legs and arms to power the move. Bend your knees.

FIRST AID MATERIALS

All workplaces, leisure centers, homes, and cars should have first aid kits. The kits for workplaces or public places must conform to legal requirements and be clearly marked and easily accessible. For home or the car, you can either buy a kit or put together first aid items yourself and keep them in a clean, waterproof container. Any first aid kit must be kept in a dry place, and it should be checked and replenished regularly.

The items shown on these pages form the basis of a first aid kit for the home. You may wish to add pain-relief tablets such as acetaminophen or ibuprofen.

STERILE DRESSINGS

Wound dressings

The most useful dressings consist of a dressing pad attached to a roller bandage, and are sealed in a protective wrapping. They are easy to apply, so they are ideal in an emergency. Various sizes are available. Individual sterile dressing pads that can be secured with tape or bandages are also available. Dressings with a nonstick suface are useful.

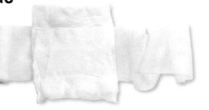

STERILE WOUND DRESSING

STERILE GAUZE PAD

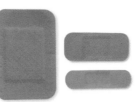

STERILE EYE PAD

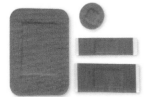

FABRIC BANDAGES

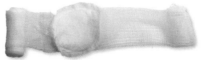

WATERPROOF BANDAGES

NOVELTY BANDAGES FOR CHILDREN

Adhesive dressings or bandages

These are applied to small cuts and abrasions and are made of fabric or waterproof plastic. Use hypoallergenic bandages for anyone who is allergic to the adhesive in regular ones. Special gel bandages can protect blisters.

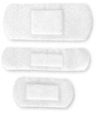

CLEAR BANDAGES

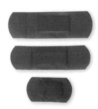

BLUE CATERING BANDAGES

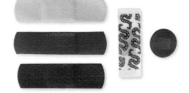

GEL BLISTER BANDAGE

« FIRST AID MATERIALS

BANDAGES

Rollers

These items are used to give support to injured joints, secure dressings in place, maintain pressure on wounds, and limit swelling.

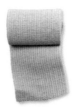 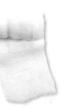 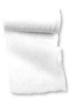

| CONFORMING ELASTIC ROLLER | GAUZE WRAP ROLLER | ELASTIC ROLLER | SELF-ADHESIVE ROLLER |

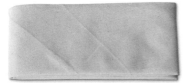

FOLDED TRIANGULAR BANDAGE

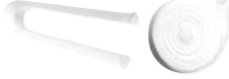

GAUZE TUBULAR BANDAGE AND APPLICATOR

Triangular bandages

Made of cloth, these items can be used folded as bandages or slings. If they are sterile and individually wrapped, they may also be used as dressings for large wounds and burns.

Gauze tubular bandages

Gauze tubular bandages are used with an applicator to secure dressings on fingers and toes. Elasticated tubular bandages are sometimes used to support injured joints such as the knee or elbow.

PROTECTIVE ITEMS

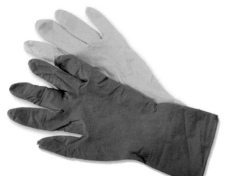

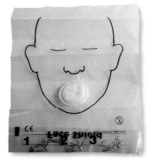

FACE SHIELD

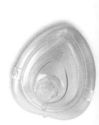

POCKET MASK

Disposable gloves

Wear gloves, if available, whenever you dress wounds or when you handle body fluids or other waste materials. Use latex-free gloves because some people are allergic to latex.

Protection from infection in CPR

You can use a plastic face shield or a pocket mask to protect you and the casualty from cross infections when giving rescue breaths.

ADDITIONAL ITEMS

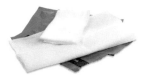 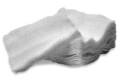 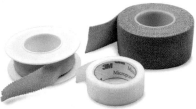

Cleansing wipes
Alcohol-free wipes can be used to clean skin around wounds.

Gauze pads
Use these pads as dressings, as padding, or as swabs to clean around wounds.

Adhesive tape
Use tape to secure dressings or the loose ends of bandages. If the casualty is allergic to the adhesive on the tape, use a hypoallergenic tape.

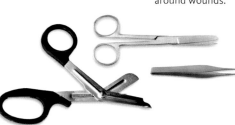

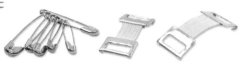

Scissors, shears, and tweezers
Choose items that are blunt-ended so that they will not cause injuries. Use shears to cut clothing.

Pins and clips
Use these to secure the ends of bandages.

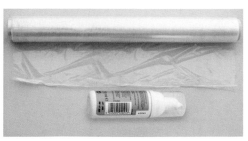

Useful items
Plastic wrap or clean plastic bags can be used to dress burns and scalds. Nonstick dressings can be kept for larger wounds. Keep alcohol gel to clean your hands when no water is available.

For use outdoors
A blanket can protect a casualty from cold. Survival bags are very compact and will keep a person warm and dry in an emergency. A flashlight helps visibility, and a whistle can be used to summon help.

BASIC MATERIALS FOR A GENERAL FIRST AID KIT

- Easily identifiable watertight box
- 20 adhesive bandages in assorted sizes
- Six medium sterile dressings
- Two large sterile dressings
- One sterile eye pad
- Six triangular bandages

- Six safety pins
- Disposable gloves
- Two roller bandages
- Scissors
- Tweezers
- Alcohol-free wound cleansing wipes
- Adhesive tape

- Plastic face shield or pocket mask
- Notepad and pencil
- Alcohol gel (hand sanitizer)

Other useful items:
- Blanket, survival bag, flashlight, whistle
- Flares, warning triangles, and high visibility jacket to keep in the car

DRESSINGS

Always cover a wound with a dressing because this helps prevent infection. With severe bleeding, pressure dressings are used to help the blood-clotting process by exerting pressure on the wound.

Use a prepacked sterile wound dressing with a bandage attached (opposite) whenever possible.

If no such dressing is available, use a sterile pad. Alternatively, any clean, nonfluffy material can be used to improvize a dressing (p.240). Protect small cuts with an adhesive dressing (p.241).

RULES FOR USING DRESSINGS

When handling or applying a dressing, there are a number of rules to follow. These enable you to apply dressings correctly; they also protect the casualty and yourself from cross infection.

- **Always put on disposable gloves,** if they are available, before handling any dressing.
- **Cover the wound** with a dressing that extends beyond the wound's edges.
- **Hold the edge of the dressing,** keeping your fingers well away from the area that will be in contact with the wound.
- **Place the dressing** directly on top of the wound; do not slide it on from the side.
- **Remove and replace** any dressing that slips out of position.

- **If you only have one sterile dressing,** use this to cover the wound, and put other clean materials on top of it.
- **If blood seeps through** the dressing, do not remove it; instead, place another dressing over the top. If blood seeps through the second dressing, remove both dressings completely and then apply a fresh dressing, making sure that you put pressure on the bleeding point.
- **After treating a wound,** dispose of gloves, used dressings, and soiled items in a suitable plastic bag, such as a red biohazard bag. Keep disposable gloves on until you have finished handling any materials that may be contaminated, then put them in the bag.

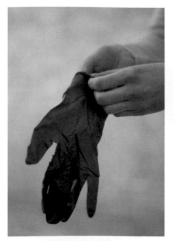

WEAR DISPOSABLE GLOVES

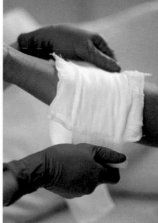

USE DRESSING LARGER THAN WOUND

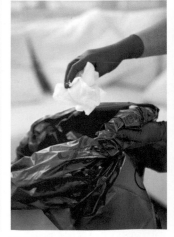

DISPOSE OF WASTE

HOW TO APPLY A STERILE WOUND DRESSING

This type of dressing consists of a dressing pad attached to a elastic bandage. The pad is a piece of gauze backed by a layer of cotton wool or padding.

Sterile dressings are available individually wrapped in various sizes. They are sealed in protective wrappings to keep them sterile. Once the seal on this type of dressing has been broken, the dressing is no longer sterile.

CAUTION

- If the dressing slips out of place, remove it and apply a new dressing.
- Take care not to impair the circulation beyond the dressing (p.243).

WHAT TO DO

1 **Break the seal** and remove the wrapping. Unwind some of the bandage, taking care not to drop the roll or touch the dressing pad.

2 **Unfold the dressing pad,** and lay it directly on the wound. Hold the bandage on each side of the pad as you place it over the wound.

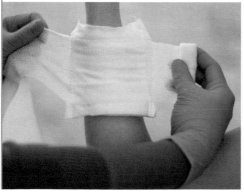

3 **Wind the short end** of the bandage once around the limb and the pad to secure the dressing.

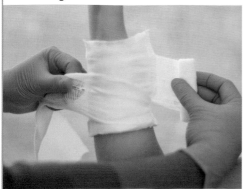

4 **Wind the other end** (head) of the bandage around the limb to cover the whole pad. Leave the short end of the bandage hanging free.

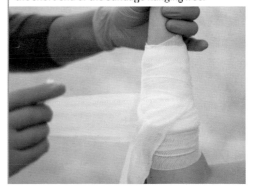

5 **To secure the bandage,** tie the ends in a square knot (p.250), directly over the pad to maintain firm pressure on the wound.

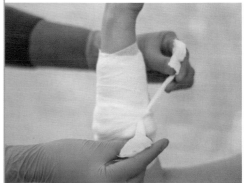

6 **Once you have secured the bandage,** check the circulation in the limb beyond it (p.243). Loosen the bandage if it is too tight, then reapply. Recheck every ten minutes.

« DRESSINGS

STERILE PAD AND GAUZE DRESSINGS

If there is no sterile wound dressing with a bandage available, use a sterile pad or make a pad with pieces of gauze. Make sure the pad is large enough to extend well beyond the edges of the wound. Hold the dressing face down; never touch the part of the dressing that will be in contact with a wound. Secure the dressing with tape. If you need to maintain pressure to control bleeding, use a bandage.

WHAT TO DO

1 Holding the dressing or pad by the edges, place it directly onto the wound.

2 Secure the pad with adhesive tape or a roller bandage.

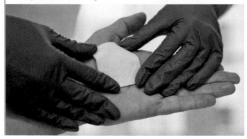
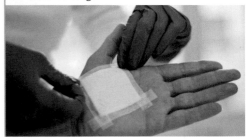

IMPROVISED DRESSINGS

If you have no suitable dressings, any clean nonfluffy material can be used in an emergency. If using a piece of folded cloth, hold it by its edges, unfold it, then refold it so that the clean inner side can be placed against the wound.

WHAT TO DO

1 Hold the material by the edges. Open it out and refold it so that the inner surface faces outward.

2 Place the cloth pad directly on the wound. If necessary, cover the pad with more material.

3 Secure the pad with a bandage or a clean strip of cloth, such as a scarf. Tie the ends in a square knot (p.250).

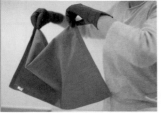
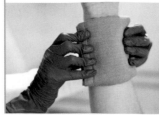
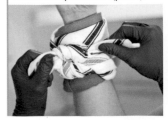

ADHESIVE BANDAGES

These are useful for dressing small cuts and scrapes. They consist of a gauze or cellulose pad and an adhesive backing, and are often wrapped singly in sterile packs. There are several sizes available, and special shapes for use on fingertips, heels, and elbows; some types are waterproof. Blister bandages have an oval cushioned pad. People who work with food must cover any wounds with waterproof adhesive bandages.

CAUTION

- Check that the casualty is not allergic to the adhesive dressings. If he is, use hypoallergenic tape or a pad and bandage.

WHAT TO DO

1 Clean and dry the skin around the wound. Unwrap the adhesive bandage and hold it by the protective strips over the backing, with the pad side facing downward.

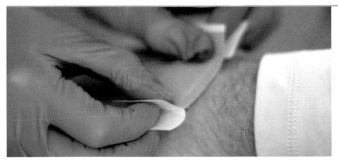

2 Peel back the strips to expose the pad, but do not remove them. Without touching the pad surface, place the pad on the wound.

3 Carefully pull away the protective strips, then press down the edges of the bandage.

COLD COMPRESSES

Cooling an injury such as a bruise or sprain can reduce swelling and pain. There are two types of compress: cold pads, which are made from material dampened with cold water, and ice packs. An ice pack can be made using crushed ice and a small amount of water sealed in a plastic bag, or packages of frozen peas or other small vegetables.

CAUTION

- To prevent cold injuries, always wrap an ice pack in a cloth. Do not leave it on the skin for more than ten minutes at a time.

COLD PAD

1 Soak a clean washcloth or towel in cold water. Wring it out lightly and fold it into a pad. Hold it firmly against the injury (right).

2 Resoak the pad in cold water every few minutes to keep it cold. Cool the injury for at least ten minutes.

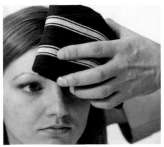

USING A COLD COMPRESS

ICE PACK

1 Partly fill a plastic bag with crushed ice, or use a pack of frozen vegetables. Wrap the bag in a dry cloth.

2 Hold the pack firmly on the area (left). Cool the injury for no more than ten minutes at a time, removing the pack for five-minute periods.

241

PRINCIPLES OF BANDAGING

There are a number of different first aid uses for bandages: they can be used to secure dressings, control bleeding, support and immobilize limbs, and reduce swelling in an injured limb. There are three main types of bandages. Roller bandages secure dressings and support injured limbs. Tubular bandages hold dressings on fingers or toes, or support injured joints. Triangular bandages can be used as large dressings, as slings, to secure dressings, or to immobilize limbs. If you have no bandage available, you can improvise from everyday items; for example, you can fold a square of fabric, such as a headscarf, diagonally to make a triangular bandage (p.249).

RULES FOR APPLYING A BANDAGE

- **Reassure the casualty** before applying a bandage and explain clearly what you are going to do.
- **Help the casualty** sit or lie down in a comfortable position.

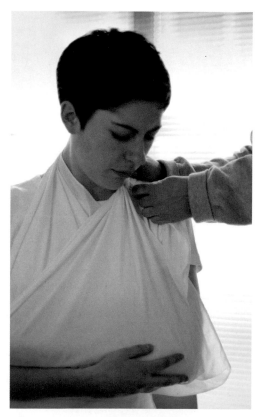

- **Support the injured part** of the body while you are working on it. Ask the casualty or a helper to do this.
- **Work from the front** of the casualty, and from the injured side where possible.
- **Pass the bandages** through the body's natural hollows at the ankles, knees, waist, and neck, then slide them into position by easing them back and forth under the body.
- **Apply bandages firmly,** but not so tightly that they interfere with circulation to the area beyond the bandage (opposite).
- **Fingers or toes** should be left exposed, if possible, so that you can check the circulation afterward.
- **Use square knots** to tie bandages (p.250). Ensure that the knots do not cause discomfort, and do not tie the knot over a bony area. Tuck loose ends under a knot if possible, to provide additional padding.
- **Check the circulation** in the area beyond the bandage (opposite) every ten minutes once it is secured. If necessary, unroll the bandage until the blood supply returns, and reapply it more loosely.

| **SEE ALSO** Roller bandages **pp.244–47** | Triangular bandages **p.249** | Tubular gauze bandages **p.248**

IMMOBILIZING A LIMB

When applying bandages to immobilize a limb you also need to use soft, bulky material, such as towels or clothing, as padding. Place the padding between the legs, or between an arm and the body, so that the bandaging does not displace broken bones or press bony areas against each other. Use folded triangular bandages and tie them at intervals along the limb, avoiding the injury site. Secure with square knots (p.250) tied on the uninjured side. If both sides of the body are injured, tie knots in the middle or where there is least chance of causing further damage.

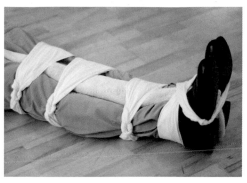
TIE KNOTS ON THE UNINJURED SIDE, NEVER OVER JOINT OR FRACTURE

CHECKING CIRCULATION AFTER BANDAGING

When bandaging a limb or applying a sling, you must check the circulation in the hand or foot immediately after you have finished bandaging, and every ten minutes thereafter. These checks are essential because limbs can swell after an injury, and a bandage can rapidly become too tight and restrict blood circulation to the area beyond it. If this occurs, you need to undo the bandage and reapply it more loosely.

RECOGNITION

If circulation is impaired there may be:

- A swollen and congested limb
- Blue skin with prominent veins
- A feeling that the skin is painfully distended.

Later there may be:

- Pale, waxy skin
- Skin cold to touch
- Numbness and tingling followed by severe pain
- Inability to move affected fingers or toes.

WHAT TO DO

1 **Press one of the nails** or the skin beyond the bandage, for five seconds until it turns pale, then release the pressure. If the color does not return within two seconds, the bandage is too tight.

2 **Loosen a tight bandage** by unrolling enough turns for warmth and color to return to the skin. The casualty may feel a tingling sensation. If necessary, loosen and reapply the bandage. Recheck every ten minutes.

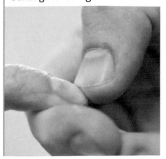

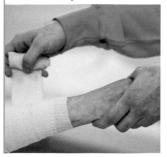

ROLLER BANDAGES

These bandages are made of cotton, gauze, elastic fabric, or linen and are wrapped around the injured part of the body in spiral turns. There are three main types of roller bandage.

- **Open-weave bandages,** often made of gauze, are used to hold dressings in place. Their loose weave allows good ventilation, but they cannot be used to exert direct pressure on the wound to control bleeding or to provide support to joints.
- **Self-adhesive support bandages** are used to support muscle (and joint) injuries and do not need pins or clips.
- **Elastic bandages** are used to give firm, even support to injured joints.

SECURING ROLLER BANDAGES

There are several ways to fasten the end of a roller bandage. Safety pins or adhesive tape are usually included in first aid kits. Some bandage packs may contain bandage clips. If you do not have any of these, a simple tuck should keep the bandage end in place.

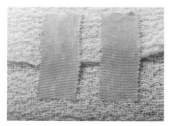

Adhesive tape
The ends of bandages can be folded under and then stuck down with small strips of adhesive tape.

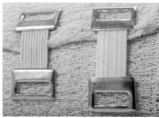

Bandage clip
Metal clips are sometimes supplied with elastic roller bandages for securing the ends.

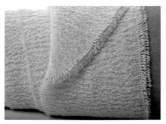

Tucking in the end
If you have no fastening, secure the bandage by passing the end around the limb once and tucking it in.

Safety pin
These pins can secure all types of roller bandage. Fold the end of the bandage under, then put your finger under the bandage to prevent injury as you insert the pin (right). Make sure that, once fastened, the pin lies flat (far right).

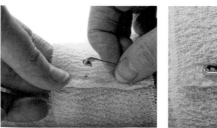

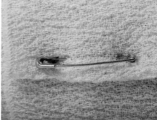

CHOOSING THE CORRECT SIZE OF BANDAGE

Before applying a roller bandage, check that it is tightly rolled and of a suitable width for the injured area. Small areas such as fingers require narrow bandages of approximately 1 in (2.5 cm) wide, while wider bandages of 4–6 in (10–15 cm) are more suitable for large areas such as legs. It is better for a roller bandage to be too wide than too narrow. Smaller sizes may be needed for a child.

APPLYING A ROLLER BANDAGE

Follow the general rules below when applying a roller bandage to an injury.

- **Keep the rolled** part of the bandage (the "head") uppermost as you work. (The unrolled short end is called the "tail.")
- **Position yourself** in front of the casualty, on the injured side.
- **Support the injured** part while you apply the bandage.

CAUTION

- Once you have applied the bandage, check the circulation in the limb beyond it (p.243). This is especially important if you are applying an elastic bandage because these mold to the shape of the limb and therefore may become tighter if the limb swells.

WHAT TO DO

1 **Place the tail of the bandage** below the injury. Working from the inside of the limb outward, make two straight turns with the bandage to anchor the tail in place.

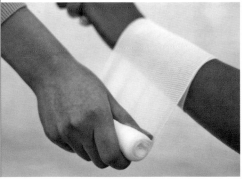

2 **Wind the bandage in spiraling turns** working from the inner to the outer side of the limb, and work up the limb. Cover one half to two-thirds of the previous layer of bandage with each new turn.

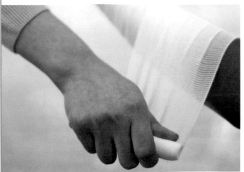

3 **Finish with one straight turn.** If the bandage is too short, apply another one in the same way so that the injured area is covered.

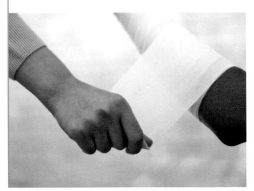

4 **Secure the end of the bandage,** then check the circulation beyond the bandage (p.243). If necessary, unroll the bandage until the blood supply returns, and reapply it more loosely. Recheck every ten minutes.

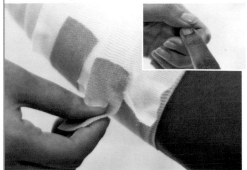

« ROLLER BANDAGES

ELBOW AND KNEE BANDAGES

Roller bandages can be used on elbows and knees to support soft tissue injuries such as strains or sprains. To ensure that there is effective support, flex the joint slightly, then apply the bandage in figure-eight turns rather than the standard spiraling turns (p.245). Work from the inside to the outside of the upper surface of the joint. Extend the bandaging far enough on either side of the joint to exert an even pressure.

WHAT TO DO

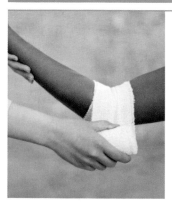

1 **Support the injured limb** in a comfortable position for the casualty, with the joint partially flexed. Place the tail of the bandage on the inner side of the joint. Pass the bandage over and around to the outside of the joint. Make one-and-a-half turns, so that the tail end of the bandage is fixed and the joint is covered.

2 **Pass the bandage** to the inner side of the limb, just above the joint. Make a turn around the limb, covering the upper half of the bandage from the first turn.

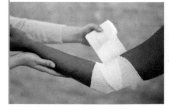

3 **Pass the bandage** from the inner side of the upper limb to just below the joint. Make one diagonal turn below the elbow joint to cover the lower half of the bandaging from the first straight turn.

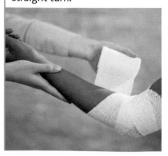

4 **Continue to bandage** diagonally above and below the joint in a figure-eight. Increase the bandaged area by covering about two-thirds of the previous turn with each new layer.

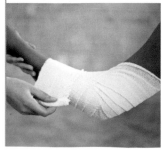

5 **To finish bandaging** the joint, make two straight turns around the limb, then secure the end of the bandage (p.244). Check the circulation beyond the bandage as soon as you have finished, then recheck every ten minutes (p.243). If necessary, unroll the bandage and reapply more loosely.

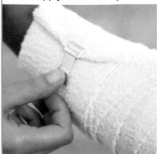

HAND BANDAGES

A elastic bandage may be applied to hold dressings in place on a hand, or to support a wrist in soft tissue injuries. A support bandage should extend well beyond the injury site to provide pressure over the entire injured area.

WHAT TO DO

1 **Place the tail** of the bandage on the inner side of the wrist, by the base of the thumb. Make two straight turns around the wrist.

2 **Working from the inner side** of the wrist, pass the bandage diagonally across the back of the hand to the nail of the little finger, and across the front of the casualty's fingers.

3 **Pass the bandage** diagonally across the back of the hand to the outer side of the wrist. Take the bandage under the wrist. Then repeat the diagonal over the back of the hand.

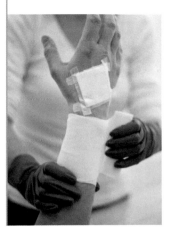

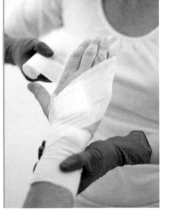

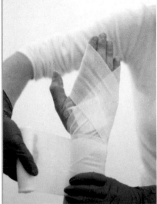

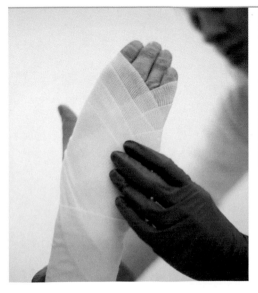

4 **Repeat the sequence** of figure-eight turns. Extend the bandaging by covering about two-thirds of the bandage from the previous turn with each new layer. When the hand is completely covered, finish with two straight turns around the wrist.

5 **Secure the end** (p.244). As soon as you have finished, check the circulation beyond the bandage (p.243), then recheck every ten minutes. If necessary, unroll the bandage until the blood supply returns and reapply it more loosely.

TUBULAR GAUZE BANDAGES

These bandages are rolls of seamless, tubular fabric. The tubular gauze bandage is used with a special applicator, which is supplied with the bandage. It is suitable for holding dressings in place on a finger or toe, but not to control bleeding.

APPLYING A TUBULAR GAUZE

1 **Cut a piece of tubular gauze** about two-and-a-half times the length of the injured finger. Push the whole length of the tubular gauze onto the applicator, then gently slide the applicator over the casualty's finger.

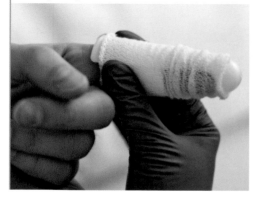

3 **While still holding the gauze** at the base of the finger, gently push the applicator back over the finger to apply a second layer of gauze. Once the gauze has been applied, remove the applicator from the finger.

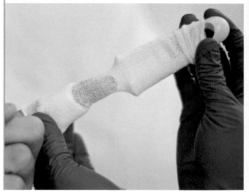

2 **Holding the end of the gauze** on the finger, pull the applicator slightly beyond the fingertip to leave a gauze layer on the finger. Twist the applicator twice to seal the bandage over the end of the finger.

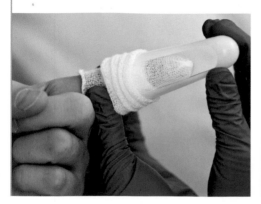

4 **Secure the gauze** at the base of the finger with adhesive tape. Check the circulation to the finger immediately (p.243) and then again every ten minutes. Ask the casualty if the finger feels cold or tingly. If it does, remove the gauze and reapply it more loosely.

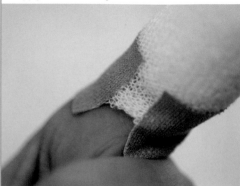

TRIANGULAR BANDAGES

This type of bandage may be supplied in a sterile pack as part of a first aid kit. You can also make one by cutting or folding a square yard of sturdy fabric diagonally in half. The bandage can be used in the following three ways.

- **Folded as a broad-fold bandage** or narrow-fold bandage (right) to immobilize and support a limb or to secure a splint or bulky dressing.
- **Opened to form a sling,** or to hold a hand, foot, or scalp dressing in place.
- **From a sterile pack,** folded into a pad and used as a sterile dressing.

MAKING A BROAD-FOLD BANDAGE

1 **Open out a triangular bandage** and lay it flat on a clean surface. Fold the bandage in half horizontally, so that the point of the triangle touches the center of the base.

2 **Fold the bandage in half again** in the same direction, so that the first folded edge touches the base. The bandage should now form a broad strip.

MAKING A NARROW-FOLD BANDAGE

1 **Fold a triangular bandage** to make a broad-fold bandage (above).

2 **Fold the bandage horizontally** in half again. It should form a long, narrow, thick strip of material.

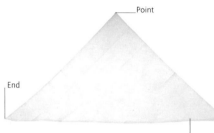

Point

End

OPEN TRIANGULAR BANDAGE | Base

STORING A TRIANGULAR BANDAGE

Keep triangular bandages in their packs so that they remain sterile until you need them. Alternatively, fold them as shown (right) so that they are ready for use as a pad or bandage, or can be shaken open.

1 **Start by folding** the triangle into a narrow-fold bandage (above). Bring the two ends of the bandage into the center.

2 **Continue folding** the ends into the center until the bandage is a convenient size for storing. Keep the bandage in a dry place.

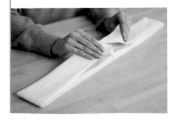

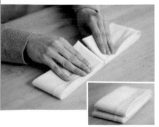

SQUARE KNOTS

When securing a triangular bandage, always use a square knot. It is secure and will not slip, it is easy to untie, and it lies flat, so it is more comfortable for the casualty. Avoid tying the knot around or directly over the injury, since this may cause discomfort.

TYING AND UNTYING A SQUARE KNOT

1 Pass the left end of the bandage (dark) over and under the right end (light).

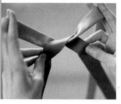

2 Lift both ends of the bandage above the rest of the material.

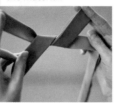

3 Pass the end in your right hand (dark) over and under the left end (light).

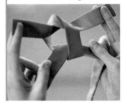

4 Pull the ends to tighten the knot, then tuck them under the bandage.

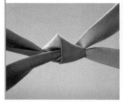

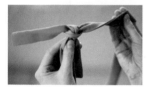

Untying a square knot
Pull one end and one piece of bandage from the same side of the knot firmly so that the piece of bandage straightens. Hold the knot and pull the straightened end through it.

HAND AND FOOT COVER

An open triangular bandage can be used to hold a dressing in place on a hand or foot, but it will not provide enough pressure to control bleeding. The method for covering a hand (right) can also be used for a foot, with the bandage ends tied at the ankle.

1 Lay the bandage flat. Place the casualty's hand on the bandage, fingers toward the point. Fold the point over the hand.

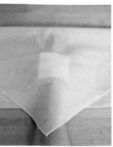

2 Cross the ends over the hand, and pass around the wrist in opposite directions. Tie the ends in a square knot (above).

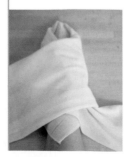

3 Pull the point gently to tighten the bandage. Fold the point up over the knot and tuck it in.

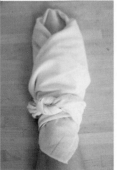

ARM SLING

An arm sling holds the forearm in a slightly raised or horizontal position. It provides support for an injured upper arm, wrist, or forearm, on a casualty whose elbow can be bent, or to immobilize the arm for a rib fracture (p.154). An elevation sling (p.252) is used to keep the forearm and hand raised in a higher position.

WHAT TO DO

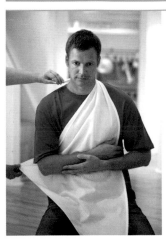

1 Ensure that the injured arm is supported with the hand slightly higher than the elbow. Fold the base of the bandage under to form a hem. Place the bandage with the base parallel to the casualty's body and level with his little fingernail. Slide the upper end under the injured arm and pull it around the neck to the opposite shoulder.

2 Fold the lower end of the bandage up over the forearm and bring it to meet the upper end at the shoulder.

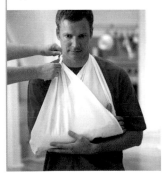

3 Tie a square knot (opposite) on the injured side, at the hollow above the casualty's collarbone. Tuck both free ends of the bandage under the knot to pad it. Adjust the sling so that the front edge supports the hand—it should extend to the top of the casualty's little finger.

4 Hold the point of the bandage beyond the elbow and twist it until the fabric fits the elbow snugly, then tuck it in or knot it. Alternatively, if you have a safety pin, fold the fabric and fasten it to the front.

5 Bind the finished sling to the body with another triangular bandage or swathe. As soon as you have finished, check the circulation in the fingers (p.243). Recheck every ten minutes. If necessary, loosen and reapply the bandages and sling.

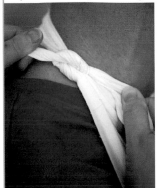

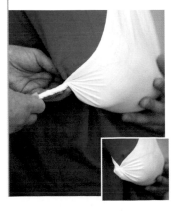

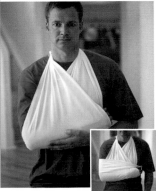

ELEVATION SLING

This form of sling supports the forearm and hand in a raised position, with the fingertips touching the casualty's shoulder. In this way, an elevation sling helps control bleeding from wounds in the forearm or hand, to minimize swelling. An elevation sling is also used to support the arm in the case of an injured hand.

WHAT TO DO

1 **Ask the casualty** to support his injured arm across his chest, with the fingers resting on the opposite shoulder.

2 **Place the bandage** over his body, with one end over the shoulder on the uninjured side. Hold the point just beyond his elbow.

3 **Ask the casualty** to let go of his injured arm while you tuck the base of the bandage under his hand, forearm, and elbow.

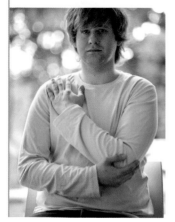 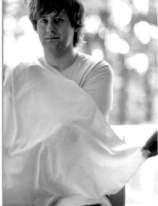 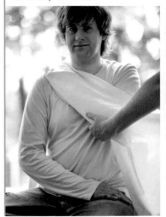

4 **Bring the lower end** of the bandage up diagonally across his back, to meet the other end at his shoulder.

5 **Tie the ends** in a square knot (p.250) at the hollow above the casualty's collarbone. Tuck ends under the knot to pad it.

6 **Twist the point** until the bandage fits closely around the casualty's elbow. Tuck the point in just above his elbow to secure it. If you have a safety pin, fold the fabric over the elbow and fasten the point at the corner. Check the circulation in the thumb every ten minutes (p.243); loosen and reapply if necessary.

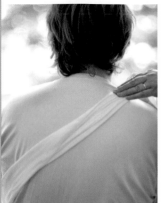 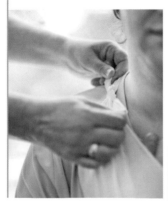 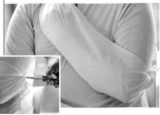

IMPROVISED SLINGS

If you need to support a casualty's injured arm but do not have a triangular bandage available, you can make a sling by using a square yard (just under one square meter) of any strong cloth (p.249). You can also improvise by using an item of the casualty's clothing (below). Check circulation after applying support (p.243) and recheck every ten minutes.

CAUTION

If you suspect that the forearm is broken, use a cloth sling or a jacket corner to provide support. Do not use any other improvised sling: it will not provide enough support.

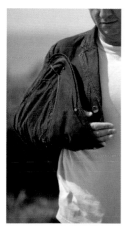

Jacket corner
Undo the casualty's jacket. Fold the lower edge on the injured side up over his arm. Secure the corner of the hem to the jacket breast with a large safety pin. Tuck and pin the excess material closely around the elbow.

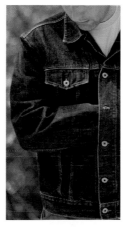

Button-up jacket
Undo one button of a jacket or coat (or waistcoat). Place the hand of the injured arm inside the garment at the gap formed by the unfastened button. Advise the casualty to rest his wrist on the button just beneath the gap.

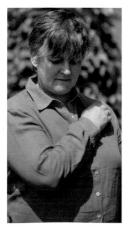

Long-sleeved shirt
Lay the injured arm across the casualty's chest. Pin the cuff of the sleeve to the breast of the shirt. To improvise an elevation sling (opposite), pin the sleeve at the casualty's opposite shoulder, to keep her arm raised.

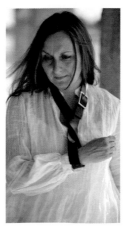

Belt or thin garment
Use a belt, a tie, a pair of suspenders, or panty hose to make a "collar-and-cuff" support. Fasten the item to form a loop. Place it over the casualty's head, then twist it once to form a smaller loop at the front. Place the casualty's hand into the loop.

12

This chapter is designed as a user-friendly quick-reference guide to first aid treatment for casualties with serious illnesses or injuries, but it is not a substitute for certified CPR and first aid training. It begins with an action plan to help identify first aid priorities, using the primary survey (pp.44–45) followed by the secondary survey (pp.46–48) where appropriate.

The chapter goes on to show how to treat unconscious casualties, whose care always takes priority over that of less seriously injured casualties. In addition, there is step-by-step essential first aid for potentially life-threatening illnesses and injuries that benefit from immediate first aid. These include asthma, stroke, severe bleeding, shock, heart attack, burns, broken bones, and spinal injuries. Each condition is described in more detail in the main part of the book and cross-referenced here so it can easily be found if you need further advice.

AIMS AND OBJECTIVES

- To protect yourself from danger and make the area safe.
- To assess the situation quickly and calmly and summon appropriate help.
- To assist casualties and provide necessary treatment with the help of bystanders.
- To **call 911 for emergency help** if you suspect a serious illness or injury.
- To be aware of your own needs.

**EMERGENCY
FIRST AID**

ACTION IN AN EMERGENCY

Assess the casualty using the primary survey (pp.44–45). Identify life-threatening conditions and once these are managed, carry out a secondary survey (pp.46–48).

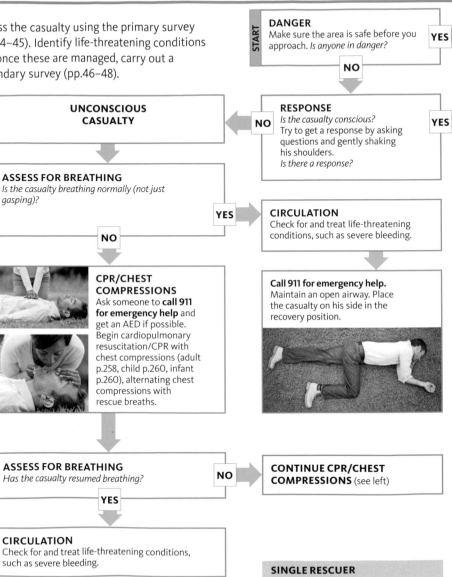

START

DANGER
Make sure the area is safe before you approach. *Is anyone in danger?* **YES**

NO

RESPONSE
Is the casualty conscious?
Try to get a response by asking questions and gently shaking his shoulders.
Is there a response? **YES**

NO

UNCONSCIOUS CASUALTY

ASSESS FOR BREATHING
Is the casualty breathing normally (not just gasping)?

YES

CIRCULATION
Check for and treat life-threatening conditions, such as severe bleeding.

NO

CPR/CHEST COMPRESSIONS
Ask someone to **call 911 for emergency help** and get an AED if possible. Begin cardiopulmonary resuscitation/CPR with chest compressions (adult p.258, child p.260, infant p.260), alternating chest compressions with rescue breaths.

Call 911 for emergency help.
Maintain an open airway. Place the casualty on his side in the recovery position.

ASSESS FOR BREATHING
Has the casualty resumed breathing?

NO

CONTINUE CPR/CHEST COMPRESSIONS (see left)

YES

CIRCULATION
Check for and treat life-threatening conditions, such as severe bleeding.

COMPRESSION-ONLY CPR

Give chest compressions only if you have not had formal training in CPR or you are unwilling or unable to give rescue breaths. The 911 dispatcher will give instructions for compression-only CPR.

SINGLE RESCUER

If you are alone, **call 911 for emergency help**, then commence CPR (adult p.258). If the casualty is a child or an infant, give chest compressions and rescue breaths (CPR) for two minutes (child p.260, infant p.260). **Call 911 for emergency help**, then continue CPR.

If it is not safe, do not approach.
Call 911 for emergency help.

CONSCIOUS CASUALTY

AIRWAY AND BREATHING

If a person is conscious and alert, it follows that her airway is open and clear. Breathing may be fast, slow, easy, or difficult. Assess and treat any difficulty found.

CIRCULATION

Are there life-threatening conditions, such as severe bleeding or heart attack?

YES

TREAT LIFE-THREATENING INJURIES OR ILLNESS.

Call 911 for emergency help. Monitor and record casualty's level of response, breathing, and pulse while you wait for help to arrive.

NO

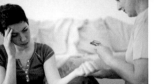

CARRY OUT A SECONDARY SURVEY

Assess the level of consciousness using the AVPU scale (p.52) and carry out a head-to-toe survey to check for signs of illness or injury.

Call for appropriate help. **Call 911 for emergency help** if you suspect serious injury or illness. Monitor and record casualty's level of response, breathing, and pulse while you wait for help to arrive.

CPR FOR AN ADULT

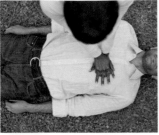

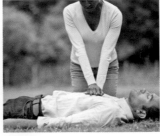

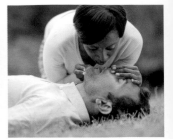

1 POSITION HANDS ON CHEST

Place one hand on the center of the casualty's chest. Place the heel of your other hand on top of the first and interlock your fingers, but keep your fingers off the casualty's ribs.

2 GIVE 30 CHEST COMPRESSIONS

Lean directly over the casualty's chest and press down vertically at least 2 in (5 cm). Release the pressure, but do not remove your hands. Give 30 compressions at a rate of at least 100 per minute.

3 BEGIN RESCUE BREATHS

Pinch the casualty's nose firmly to close the nostrils, and allow his mouth to fall open. Take a breath and seal your lips over the casualty's mouth. Blow steadily into the mouth until the chest rises—this should take about one second.

CHEST-COMPRESSION-ONLY CPR

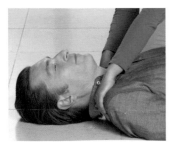

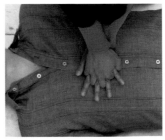

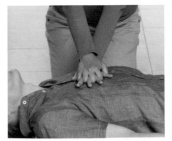

1 CHECK FOR RESPONSE

Check for a response. Gently shake the casualty's shoulders, and talk to him. Assess breathing; if casualty is not breathing or only gasping, go to the next step.

2 BEGIN CHEST COMPRESSIONS

Kneel level with the casualty's chest. Put one hand on the center of the chest and the heel of your other hand on top; interlock your fingers. Depress chest at least 2 in (5 cm), and release but keep your hands in place. Do compressions at a rate of 100 per minute.

3 CONTINUE CHEST COMPRESSIONS

Give chest compressions until emergency help arrives; the casualty shows signs of regaining consciousness, such as coughing, opening his eyes, speaking, or moving purposefully, and starts to breathe normally; or you are too exhausted to continue.

FIND OUT MORE **pp.66–69, pp.84–85**

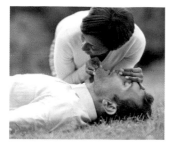

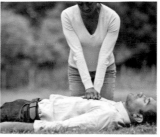

 WATCH CHEST FALL

Maintaining head tilt and chin lift, take your mouth away from the casualty's. Look along the chest and watch it fall. Repeat to give TWO rescue breaths. Repeat 30 chest compressions followed by TWO rescue breaths.

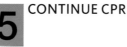 **CONTINUE CPR**

Continue CPR until emergency help arrives, the casualty starts to breathe normally, or you are too exhausted to continue. If you are unwilling or unable to give rescue breaths, you can give chest compressions alone (below).

CAUTION

- Ensure that 911 has been called.
- Obtain and use an AED as soon as possible, attaching the pads and following the instructions.
- Do not delay chest compressions until an AED becomes available.
- If the casualty vomits during CPR, roll him away from you onto his side, ensuring that his head is turned toward the floor to allow vomit to drain. Clear his mouth, then immediately roll him onto his back again and recommence CPR.

FIND OUT MORE **pp.70–71, pp.84–85**

CAUTION

- Chest-compression-only CPR is given only if you have not had formal training in CPR, or you are unwilling or unable to give rescue breaths. The dispatcher will give you instructions for chest-compression-only CPR.
- Ensure that 911 has been called.
- Use an AED as soon as possible, attaching the pads and following the instructions.
- Do not delay chest compressions until an AED becomes available.
- If there is more than one rescuer, change over every 2 minutes, with minimal interruption to chest compressions.

CPR FOR A CHILD ONE YEAR TO PUBERTY

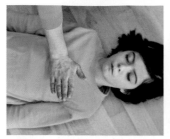

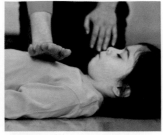

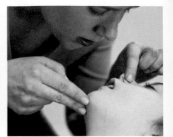

1 POSITION ONE HAND ON CHEST

Place the heel of one hand on the center of her chest, but keep your fingers off her ribs.

2 GIVE 30 CHEST COMPRESSIONS

Lean directly over the child's chest and press down vertically to about one third of its depth. Release the pressure, but do not remove your hands. Give 30 compressions at a rate of at least 100 per minute.

3 GIVE TWO RESCUE BREATHS

Pinch the nose firmly to close the nostrils. Take a breath and seal your lips over the child's mouth. Blow steadily into the mouth until the chest rises—this should take about one second.

CPR FOR AN INFANT UNDER ONE YEAR

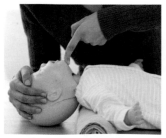

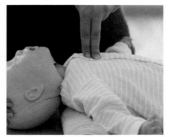

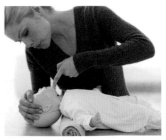

1 CHECK THAT AIRWAY IS OPEN

Place the infant on his back on a flat surface, at waist height in front of you or on the floor, with a rolled-up towel under his shoulders.

2 POSITION TWO FINGERS ON CHEST

Lean directly over the infant's chest and press down vertically to about one third of its depth— about 1½ in (4 cm). Release the pressure but do not remove your fingers. Give 30 compressions at a rate of at least 100 per minute.

3 CHECK THAT AIRWAY IS OPEN

Open the airway by putting one hand on the infant's forehead and a fingertip of the other hand under the tip of his chin, and tilting up and back as shown. Pick out any visible obstructions from mouth and nose.

FIND OUT MORE **pp.76–79**

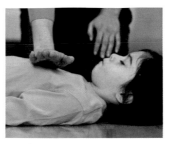

 WATCH CHEST FALL

Maintaining head tilt and chin lift, take your mouth away from the casualty's. Look along the chest and watch it fall. Repeat to give TWO rescue breaths. Repeat 30 chest compressions followed by TWO rescue breaths.

5 CONTINUE CPR

Do CPR for two minutes, then **call 911 for emergency help**. Continue CPR until emergency help arrives, the child starts to breathe normally, or you are too exhausted to continue. If you are unwilling or unable to give rescue breaths, you can give chest compressions alone.

CAUTION

- Use an AED, preferably with pediatric pads, as soon as it is available.
- If the child is large or the rescuer is small, give compressions using both hands, as for an adult (pp.258–59). Place one hand on the child's chest, cover it with your other hand, and interlock your fingers.
- If there is more than one rescuer, change over every 2 minutes, with minimal interruption to chest compressions.

FIND OUT MORE **pp.82–83**

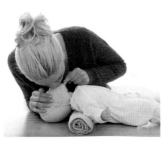

 GIVE TWO RESCUE BREATHS

Take a breath, and place your lips over the infant's mouth and nose, making sure you get a good seal. Blow steadily until the chest rises. Give TWO rescue breaths. **Call 911 for emergency help** if this has not already been done and obtain an AED if available.

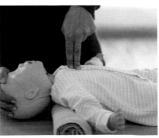

5 CONTINUE CPR

Continue CPR, alternating 30 compressions with TWO rescue breaths until emergency help takes over, the infant starts to breathe, or you are too exhausted to continue. If you are unwilling or unable to give rescue breaths, give chest compressions only.

CAUTION

- Use an AED, preferably with pediatric pads, as soon as it is available.
- If you have not had formal training in CPR or you are unwilling or unable to give rescue breaths, you can give chest compressions only. The dispatcher will give instructions for chest-compression-only CPR.
- If the infant vomits during CPR, roll him away from you onto his side, ensuring that his head is turned toward the floor to allow vomit to drain. Clear his mouth, then restart CPR as soon as possible.

HEART ATTACK

RECOGNITION

There may be:

- Vicelike chest pain, spreading to one or both arms
- Breathlessness
- Discomfort, like indigestion, in upper abdomen
- Sudden dizziness or faintness
- Sudden collapse, with no warning
- Casualty may have sense of impending doom
- Ashen skin and blueness of lips
- Rapid, weak, or irregular pulse
- Profuse sweating
- Extreme gasping for air (air hunger)

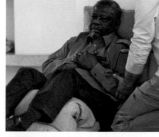

1 MAKE CASUALTY COMFORTABLE

Help the casualty into a half-sitting position. Support his head and shoulders and place cushions under his knees. Reassure the casualty.

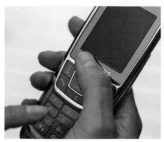

2 CALL FOR EMERGENCY HELP

Call 911 for emergency help. Tell the dispatcher that you suspect a heart attack. Call the casualty's doctor as well, if he asks you to do so.

STROKE

RECOGNITION

Use the FAST (Face—Arms—Speech—Time) guide (p.212) to assess the casualty.

- Facial weakness—casualty is unable to smile evenly
- Arm weakness—casualty may only be able to move the arm on one side of his body
- Speech problems

There may also be:

- Weakness or numbness along one side of entire body
- Sudden blurring or loss of vision
- Difficulty understanding the spoken word
- Sudden confusion
- Dizziness, unsteadiness, or a sudden fall

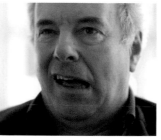

1 CHECK CASUALTY'S FACE

Keep the casualty comfortable. Ask him to smile. If he has had a stroke, he may only be able to smile on one side—the other side of his face may droop.

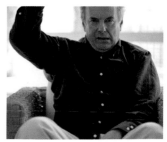

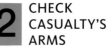

2 CHECK CASUALTY'S ARMS

Ask the casualty to raise his arms. If he has had a stroke, he may be able to lift only one arm.

FIND OUT MORE **p.211**

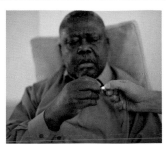

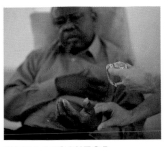

CAUTION

- Be aware of the possibility of collapse without warning.
- Do not give the casualty aspirin if he is allergic to it.
- If the casualty loses consciousness, lay him on his back, then assess breathing (p.256). Be prepared to begin CPR with compressions (pp.258–59).

 GIVE CASUALTY MEDICATION

If the casualty is fully conscious, help him take one full dose aspirin tablet (325mg); advise him to chew it slowly. If the casualty has tablets or a spray for angina, allow him to take it himself. Help him if necessary.

4 MONITOR CASUALTY

Encourage the casualty to rest. Keep any bystanders away. Monitor and record the casualty's vital signs—level of response, breathing, and pulse—until emergency help arrives.

FIND OUT MORE **pp.212–13**

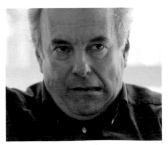

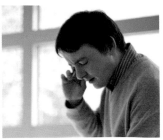

CAUTION

- Do not give the casualty anything to eat or drink; he may find it hard to swallow.
- If the person is unconscious and is not breathing normally, begin CPR with chest compressions (p.258).

 CHECK CASUALTY'S SPEECH

Ask the casualty some questions. Can he speak and/or can he understand what you are saying?

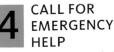 **CALL FOR EMERGENCY HELP**

Call 911 for emergency help. Tell the dispatcher that you suspect a stroke. Reassure the casualty and monitor and record his vital signs—level of response, breathing, and pulse—until help arrives.

CHOKING ADULT

RECOGNITION

Ask the casualty: "Are you choking?"

Mild obstruction:

- Difficulty in speaking, coughing and breathing

Severe obstruction:

- Inability to speak, cough, or breathe
- Eventual unconsciousness.

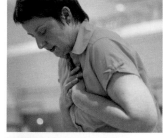

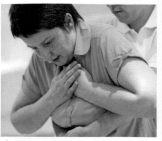

1 ENCOURAGE CASUALTY TO COUGH

If the casualty is breathing, encourage her to cough to try to remove the obstruction herself. If this fails, go to step 2.

2 GIVE ABDOMINAL THRUSTS

Stand behind the casualty. Put both arms around her, and put one fist between her navel and the bottom of her breastbone. Grasp your fist with your other hand, and pull sharply inward and upward until the object is dislodged.

CHOKING CHILD ONE YEAR TO PUBERTY

RECOGNITION

Ask the child: "Are you choking?"

Mild obstruction:

- Difficulty in speaking, coughing, and breathing

Severe obstruction:

- Inability to speak, cough, or breathe
- Eventual unconsciousness

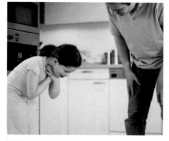

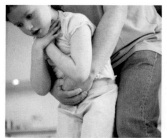

1 ENCOURAGE CHILD TO COUGH

If the child is breathing, encourage her to cough to try to remove the obstruction herself. If this fails, go to step 2.

2 GIVE ABDOMINAL THRUSTS

Stand behind the child. Put your arms around her, and put one fist between her navel and the bottom of her breastbone. Grasp your fist with your other hand, and pull sharply inward and upward until the object is expelled.

FIND OUT MORE **p.94**

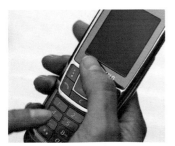

- Do not do a finger sweep when checking the mouth.
- Seek medical advice for any adult who has been given abdominal thrusts.
- If the casualty loses consciousness, assess for breathing (p.256). Be prepared to give CPR, beginning with compressions (p.258).

 CALL FOR EMERGENCY HELP

Call **911 for emergency help** if the casualty loses consciousness, then begin CPR starting with chest compressions.

FIND OUT MORE **p.95**

- Do not do a finger sweep when checking the mouth.
- Seek medical advice for any child who has been given abdominal thrusts.
- If the child loses consciousness, assess for breathing (p.256). Be prepared to begin CPR (pp.260–61).

 CALL FOR EMERGENCY HELP

Continue abdominal thrusts until the obstruction clears. If the child loses consciousness, **call 911 for emergency help,** then begin CPR starting with chest compressions.

CHOKING INFANT UNDER ONE YEAR

RECOGNITION

Mild obstruction:

- Able to cough but difficulty in breathing or making any noise

Severe obstruction:

- Inability to cough, make any noise, or breathe
- Eventual unconsciousness

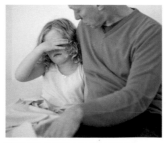

1 GIVE UP TO FIVE BACK BLOWS

If the infant is unable to cough or breathe, lay him face down along your forearm (head low), and support his body and head. Give up to five back blows between the shoulder blades with the heel of your hand.

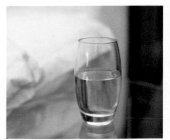

2 CHECK INFANT'S MOUTH

Turn the infant face up along your other forearm, supporting his back and head. Check the mouth. Pick out any obvious obstructions. If choking persists, proceed to step 3.

MENINGITIS

RECOGNITION

Some, but not all, of these symptoms may be present:

- Flulike illness with a high temperature
- Cold hands and feet
- Joint and/or limb pain
- Mottled or very pale skin

As infection develops:

- Neck stiffness
- Eyes become sensitive to light
- Drowsiness
- A distinctive rash of red or purple spots that look like bruises and do not fade when pressed
- In infants, a high-pitched moaning or whimpering cry, floppiness, and a tense or bulging fontanelle (soft part of the skull)

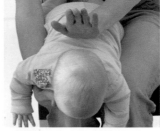

1 SEEK MEDICAL ADVICE

If you notice any signs of meningitis, such as the casualty shielding her eyes from light or a stiff neck, seek urgent medical advice.

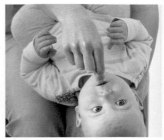

2 TREAT FEVER

Keep the casualty cool and give plenty of water to replace fluids lost through sweating. An adult may take the recommended dose of acetaminophen or ibuprofen tablets; a child may have aceta-minophen or ibuprofen syrup.

FIND OUT MORE **p.96**

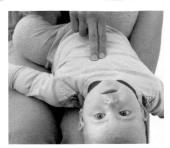

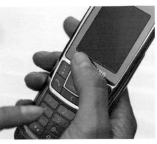

CAUTION

- Do not do a finger sweep when checking the mouth.
- Do not use abdominal thrusts on an infant.
- If the infant loses consciousness, open the airway and assess for breathing (p.256). Be prepared to begin CPR (pp.260–61).
- If a second rescuer is present, send him to **call 911 immediately,** as soon as you discover the choking infant.

 GIVE UP TO FIVE CHEST COMPRESSIONS

Place two fingertips on the lower half of the infant's breastbone, in the nipple line. Give up to five compressions. Recheck the mouth.

4 CALL FOR EMERGENCY HELP

Repeat steps 1 to 3 until the object is expelled or the infant loses consciousness. Do CPR on the unconscious infant for two minutes, **call 911 for emergency help**, then continue CPR until help arrives.

FIND OUT MORE **p.220**

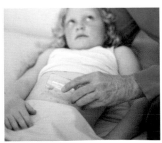

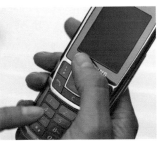

CAUTION

- If the casualty loses consciousness and is not breathing normally (p.256), begin CPR with chest compressions (pp.258–61).
- The rescuer should also seek medical advice because prophylactic antibiotics may be necessary.

 CHECK FOR SIGNS OF RASH

Check the casualty for signs of the meningitis rash: press against the rash with the side of a glass. Most rashes will fade when pressed; if you can still see the rash through the glass, it is probably meningitis.

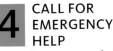 CALL FOR EMERGENCY HELP

Call 911 for emergency help if you see signs of the rash, or if medical help is delayed. Reassure the casualty. Keep her cool and monitor and record her level of response, breathing, and pulse until help arrives.

ASTHMA

- Difficulty in breathing, especially breathing out

There may be:

- Wheezing
- Difficulty speaking
- Gray-blue coloring in skin, lips, earlobes, and nailbeds

In a severe attack:

- Exhaustion and possible loss of consciousness

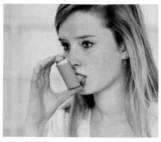

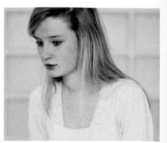

1 HELP CASUALTY USE INHALER

Keep calm and reassure the casualty. Help her find and use her inhaler (it is usually blue or white); use a spacer device if she has one. The inhaler should take effect within minutes.

2 ENCOURAGE SLOW BREATHS

Help the casualty into a comfortable breathing position; sitting slightly forward is best. Tell her to breathe slowly and deeply. A mild attack should ease within a few minutes. If it does not, ask the casualty to take another dose from her inhaler.

ANAPHYLACTIC SHOCK

There may be:

- Anxiety
- Red, blotchy skin, itchy rash, and red, itchy, watery eyes
- Swelling of hands, feet, and face
- Puffiness around the eyes
- Abdominal pain, vomiting, and diarrhea
- Difficulty breathing, ranging from tight chest to severe difficulty, which causes wheezing and gasping for air
- Swelling of tongue and throat
- A feeling of terror
- Confusion and agitation
- Signs of shock (p.270) leading to unconsciousness

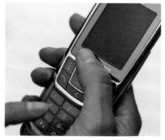

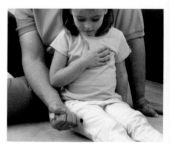

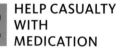

1 CALL FOR EMERGENCY HELP

Call 911 for emergency help. Ideally, ask someone to make the call while you treat the casualty. Tell the dispatcher that you suspect anaphylaxis and tell him the possible cause.

2 HELP CASUALTY WITH MEDICATION

If the casualty has an auto-injector of epinephrine, help her use it. If she is unable to take the medication, administer it yourself. Hold it in your fist, pull off the safety cap, and push the tip firmly against the casualty's thigh until it clicks (through clothing if necessary).

FIND OUT MORE **p.102**

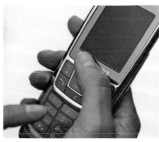
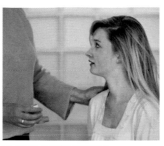

- Do not let the casualty lie down.
- Do not leave the casualty alone because the attack may quickly worsen.
- If this is a first attack and she has no medication, **call 911 for emergency help** immediately.
- If the attack worsens, the casualty may lose consciousness. Lay her on her back, then assess breathing (p.256). Be prepared to begin CPR (pp.258–61).

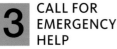

3 CALL FOR EMERGENCY HELP

Call 911 for emergency help if the inhaler has no effect, breathlessness makes talking difficult, or the casualty is becoming exhausted.

4 MONITOR CASUALTY

Monitor and record the casualty's vital signs—level of response, breathing, and pulse—until she recovers or help arrives. Help her use her inhaler as required. Advise the casualty to seek medical advice if she is concerned about the attack.

FIND OUT MORE **p.223**

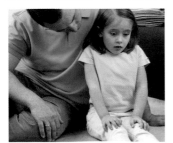
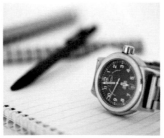

- If the casualty loses consciousness and is not breathing normally (p.256), begin CPR with chest compressions (pp.258–61).

3 MAKE CASUALTY COMFORTABLE

Reassure the casualty and help her sit in a position that eases any breathing difficulties. If she becomes very pale with a weak pulse, lay her down with legs raised as for shock.

4 MONITOR CASUALTY

Monitor and record vital signs—level of response, breathing, and pulse—until help arrives. Repeat the epinephrine dose every five minutes if there is no improvement or the casualty's symptoms return.

SEVERE EXTERNAL BLEEDING

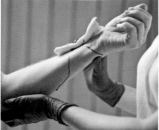

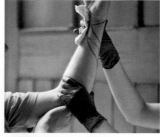

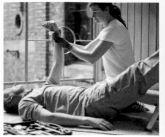

1 APPLY DIRECT PRESSURE TO WOUND

Remove or cut off any clothing over the wound if necessary. Place a sterile wound dressing or gauze pad over the wound. Apply firm pressure with your fingers or the palm of your hand.

2 RAISE AND SUPPORT INJURED PART

Maintaining pressure on the wound, raise and support the injured part so that it is above the level of the casualty's heart.

3 LAY CASUALTY DOWN

Keeping the injury high, help the casualty lie down on a blanket. Raise and support his legs to minimize the risk of shock (below).

SHOCK

RECOGNITION

- Rapid pulse
- Pale, cold, clammy skin
- Sweating

As shock develops:

- Rapid, shallow breathing
- Weak pulse
- Gray-blue skin, especially inside lips
- Weakness and giddiness
- Nausea and vomiting
- Thirst

As the brain's oxygen supply weakens:

- Restlessness
- Gasping for air
- Loss of consciousness

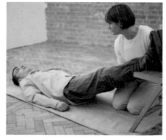

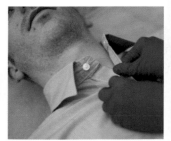

1 HELP CASUALTY LIE DOWN

Help the casualty lie down (ideally on a blanket). Raise and support his legs above the level of his heart. Treat any cause of shock, such as bleeding (above) or burns (pp.274–75).

2 LOOSEN TIGHT CLOTHING

Keep the casualty's head low. Loosen any clothing that constricts his neck, chest, and waist.

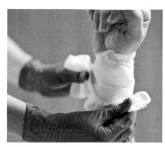

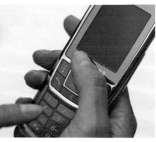

- If there is an object in the wound, apply pressure on either side of the wound to control bleeding.

- If blood seeps through the bandage, place another pad on top.

- Do not apply a tourniquet unless you have been trained and severe bleeding cannot be stopped.

- Do not give the casualty anything to eat or drink—an anesthetic may be needed.

- If the casualty loses consciousness, and is not breathing, begin CPR with chest compressions (pp.258–61).

 BANDAGE DRESSING IN PLACE

Secure a pad over the wound with a bandage. Check the circulation beyond the bandage every ten minutes. Loosen and reapply the bandage if necessary.

5 CALL FOR EMERGENCY HELP

Call 911 for emergency help. Give details of the site of the injury and the extent of the bleeding when you telephone. Monitor and record vital signs—level of response, breathing, and pulse—until emergency help arrives.

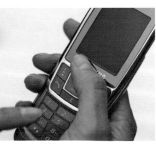

- Do not leave the casualty unattended, unless you are on your own and have to call for emergency help.

- Do not let the casualty move.

- Do not try to warm the casualty with a hot-water bottle or any other form of direct heat.

- Do not give the casualty anything to eat or drink because an anesthetic may be needed.

- If the casualty loses consciousness and is not breathing, begin CPR with chest compressions (pp.258–61).

 KEEP CASUALTY WARM

Cover the casualty with a blanket to keep him warm. Advise the casualty not to move.

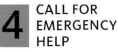 **CALL FOR EMERGENCY HELP**

Call 911 for emergency help. Give the dispatcher details about the cause of shock, if known. Monitor and record vital signs—level of response, breathing, and pulse—until help arrives.

HEAD INJURY

RECOGNITION

There may be:

- A scalp wound
- Clear fluid or watery blood from the nose or an ear (this indicates a serious underlying head injury)
- Impaired consciousness

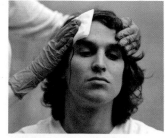

1 APPLY DIRECT PRESSURE TO ANY WOUND

Replace any displaced skin flaps over the wound. Put a sterile dressing or a clean gauze pad over the wound. Apply firm, direct pressure with your hand to control the bleeding.

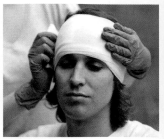

2 SECURE DRESSING WITH BANDAGE

Secure the dressing over the wound with a roller bandage to help maintain direct pressure on the injury.

SPINAL INJURY

RECOGNITION

- Can occur after a fall from a height onto the back, head, or feet

There may be:

- Pain in neck or back
- Step, irregularity, or twist in the normal curve of the spine
- Tenderness in the skin over the spine
- Weakness or loss of movement in the limbs
- Loss of sensation, or abnormal sensation
- Loss of bladder and/or bowel control
- Difficulty breathing.

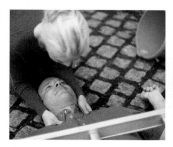

1 STEADY AND SUPPORT HEAD

Tell the casualty not to move. Sit or kneel behind his head and, resting your arms on the ground, grasp either side of the casualty's head and hold it still. Do not cover his ears.

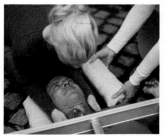

2 PLACE EXTRA SUPPORT AROUND HEAD

Continue to hold his head and ask a helper to place rolled towels, or other padding, around the casualty's neck and shoulders for extra support.

FIND OUT MORE **pp.144–45**

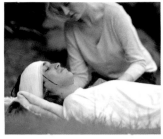

 HELP CASUALTY LIE DOWN

Help the casualty lie down, ideally on a blanket. Ensure that his head and shoulders are slightly raised. Make him as comfortable as possible.

4 MONITOR CASUALTY

Monitor and record the casualty's vital signs—level of response, breathing, and pulse. **Call 911 for emergency help** if there are any signs of severe head injury.

CAUTION

- If blood seeps through the pad, place a second one on top of the first.
- Be aware of the possibility of concussion.
- Monitor a casualty after a head injury. If he recovers initially, but deteriorates hours or days later, **call 911 for emergency help** immediately.
- If the casualty loses consciousness and is not breathing, begin CPR with chest compressions (pp.258–61).
- Always suspect the possibility of a neck (spinal) injury.

FIND OUT MORE **pp.157–59**

 CALL FOR EMERGENCY HELP

Call 911 for emergency help. If possible, ask a helper to make the call while you support the casualty's head and neck. Tell the dispatcher that a spinal injury is suspected.

4 MONITOR CASUALTY

Monitor and record the casualty's vital signs—level of response, breathing, and pulse—until help arrives.

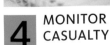

CAUTION

- Do not move the casualty unless he is in danger.
- If the casualty is unconscious, and is not breathing, begin CPR with chest compressions (pp.258–61).
- If you need to turn the casualty into the recovery position use the log-roll technique.

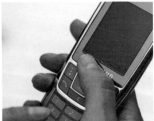

BROKEN BONES

- Distortion, swelling, and bruising at the injury site
- Pain and difficulty in moving the injured part

There may be:

- Bending, twisting, or shortening of a limb
- A wound, possibly with bone ends protruding

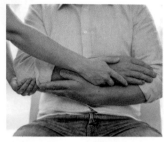

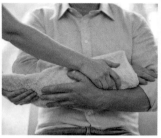

1 SUPPORT INJURED PART

Help the casualty support the affected part at the joints above and below the injury, in the most comfortable position.

2 PROTECT INJURY WITH PADDING

Place padding, such as towels or cushions, around the affected part to support it.

BURNS AND SCALDS

There may be:

- Possible areas of superficial, partial-thickness, and/or full-thickness burns
- Pain in the area of the burn
- Breathing difficulties if the airway is affected
- Swelling and blistering of the skin
- Signs of shock

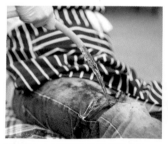

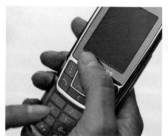

1 START TO COOL BURN

Make the casualty comfortable by helping him sit or lie down. Flood the injury with cold water; cool for at least ten minutes or until pain is relieved.

2 CALL FOR EMERGENCY HELP

Call 911 for emergency help if necessary. Tell the dispatcher that the injury is a burn and explain what caused it, and the estimated size and depth.

FIND OUT MORE **pp.136–38**

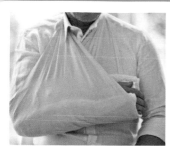

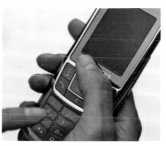

CAUTION

- Do not attempt to move an injured limb unnecessarily, or if it causes further pain.
- If there is an open wound, cover it with a sterile dressing or a clean gauze pad and bandage it in place.
- Do not give the casualty anything to eat or drink because an anesthetic may be needed.
- Do not raise an injured leg when treating a casualty for shock.

 ## SUPPORT WITH SLINGS OR BANDAGES

For extra support or if help is delayed, secure the injured part to an uninjured part of the body. For upper body injuries, use a sling; for lower limb injuries, use broad- and narrow-fold bandages. Tie knots on the uninjured side.

4 ## TAKE OR SEND CASUALTY TO THE HOSPITAL

A casualty with an arm injury could be taken by car if not in shock, but a leg injury should go by ambulance, so **call 911 for emergency help**. Treat for shock. Monitor and record the casualty's level of response, breathing, and pulse until help arrives.

FIND OUT MORE **pp.174–75**

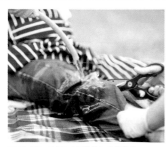

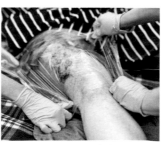

CAUTION

- Do not apply specialized dressings, lotions, or fat to a burn, but bacitracin can be used on first degree burns.
- Do not use adhesive dressings.
- Do not touch the burn or burst any blisters.
- If the burn is severe, treat the casualty for shock (p.270).
- If the burn is on the face, do not cover it. Keep cooling with water until help arrives.
- If the burn is caused by contact with chemicals, wear protective gloves and irrigate for at least 20 minutes.
- Watch the casualty for signs of smoke inhalation, such as difficulty breathing.

 ## REMOVE ANY CONSTRICTIONS

While you are cooling the burn, carefully remove any clothing or jewelry from the area before it starts to swell; a helper can do this for you. Do not remove anything that is sticking to the burn.

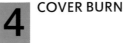 ## COVER BURN

Cover the burn with plastic wrap placed lengthwise over the injury, or use a plastic bag. Alternatively, use a sterile dressing or clean gauze pad. Monitor and record the casualty's level of response, breathing, and pulse while waiting for help.

FIRST AID REGULATIONS

First aid may be practiced in any situation where injuries or illnesses occur. In many cases, the first person on the scene is a volunteer who wants to help, rather than someone who is medically trained. However, in certain circumstances the provision of first aid, and first aid responsibilities, is defined by statutes. In the US, these regulations apply to incidents occurring in the workplace and to mass gatherings.

FIRST AID AT WORK

The Health and Safety (First Aid) Regulations of 1970 place a general duty on employers to make first aid provision for employees in case of injury or illness in the workplace. The practical aspects of this statutory duty for employers and for self-employed persons are set out in the approved code of practice, which is revised periodically to ensure that the appropriate standards are maintained. Regular occupational first aiders should make sure they are familiar with the code of practice and guidance notes.

The current code of practice stresses the aims of the first aid provision and encourages all employers to assess their organization's ability to meet those aims. The number of first aiders required in a specific workplace is dependent on the risk assessment, which should be carried out by the Compliance Safety and Health Officer in the workplace. There is a checklist (opposite) to assist in determining the number and type of first aid personnel required in a workplace. The approved code of practice also contains guidance on first aid materials, equipment, and facilities.

Comprehensive advice regarding first aid in the workplace can also be found at www.osha.gov.

ACCIDENT BOOK

An employer has the overall responsibility for an accident book, but it is the responsibility of the first aider or appointed person to look after the book.

If an employee is involved in an incident in the workplace, the following details should be recorded in the accident book.

- Date, time, and place of incident
- Name and job of the injured or ill person
- Details of the injury/illness and what first aid was given
- What happened to the person immediately afterward (for example, went home or was taken to the hospital)
- Name and signature of the first aider or person dealing with the incident

REPORTING OF INJURIES, DISEASES, AND DANGEROUS OCCURRENCES

In the event of injury or ill health at work, an employer has a legal obligation to report the incident. The Occupational Safety and Health Act (1970), under the "record-keeping rule" and the revised record-keeping rules of 2002, requires an employer to report the following:

- **Deaths**
- **Major injuries**
- **Injuries lasting more than three days**— where an employee or self-employed person is unable to perform his normal work duties
- **Injuries to members of the public** or people not at work, when they are taken from the scene of an accident to the hospital
- **Some work-related diseases**
- **Some dangerous occurrences** such as a near miss, where something happens that could have resulted in an injury

CHECKLIST FOR ASSESSMENT OF FIRST AID NEEDS

FACTORS TO CONSIDER	IMPACT ON FIRST AID PROVISION
Is your workplace low risk (for example, stores and offices)?	**The minimum provision is:** ■ An appointed person to take charge of first aid arrangements ■ A suitably stocked first aid box.
Is your workplace higher risk (for example, such as food processing or dangerous machinery)? Do your work activities involve special hazards, such as hydrofluoric acid or confined spaces?	**You should consider:** ■ Providing first aiders ■ Additional training for first aiders to deal with injuries resulting from special hazards ■ Additional first aid equipment ■ Precise siting of first aid equipment ■ Providing a first aid room ■ Informing the emergency services.
How many people are employed on site?	**Where there are small numbers of employees, the minimum provision is:** ■ An appointed person to take charge of first aid arrangements ■ A suitably stocked first aid box. Because there is still the possibility of an accident or sudden illness, you should consider providing a qualified first aider. **Where there are large numbers of employees, consider providing:** ■ First aiders ■ Additional first aid equipment ■ A first aid room.
Are there inexperienced workers on site, or employees with disabilities or special health problems?	**You should consider:** ■ Additional training for first aiders ■ Additional first aid equipment ■ Local siting of first-aid equipment. Your first aid provision should cover any work-experience trainees.
What is your record of accidents and ill health? What injuries and illness have occurred and where?	Make sure your first aid provision caters for the type of injury and illness that might occur in your workplace. Monitor accidents and ill health and review your first aid provision as appropriate.
Do you have employees who travel a lot, work remotely, or work alone?	**You should consider:** ■ Personal first aid kits ■ Personal communicators to remote workers ■ Cell phones to lone workers.
Do any of your employees work shifts or overtime?	Make sure there is adequate first aid provision at all times while people are at work.
Are the premises spread out; for example, are there several buildings on the site or multifloor buildings?	**You should consider:** ■ First aid provision in each building or on each floor.
Is your workplace remote from emergency medical services?	**You should consider:** ■ Special arrangements with the emergency services ■ Informing the emergency services of your location.
Do any of your employees work at sites occupied by other employers?	Make arrangements with other site occupiers to ensure adequate provision of first aid. A written agreement between employers is strongly recommended.
Do you have sufficient provision to cover absences of first aiders or appointed persons?	**You should consider what cover is needed for:** ■ Annual leave and other planned absences ■ Unplanned and exceptional absences.
Do members of the public visit your premises?	Under the regulations, you have no legal obligation to provide first aid for nonemployees, but the Site Contractors should be included them in your first aid provision. This is particularly relevant in workplaces that provide a service; e.g., schools, places of entertainment, fairgrounds, stores.

INDEX

ACKNOWLEDGMENTS

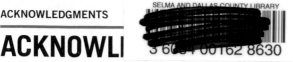

ACKNOWL[...]

AMERICAN COLLEGE OF EMERGENCY PHYSICIANS

Gina M. Piazza DO, FACEP
Medical Editor-in-Chief
Robert Heard MBA, CAE
Associate Executive Director, Membership and Education Division
Marta Foster
Director, Educational Products

AUTHORS OF 5TH EDITION

St. John Ambulance
Dr. Margaret Austin DSTJ LRCPI LRSCI LM
Deputy Chief Medical Officer

St. Andrew's First Aid
Mr. Rudy Crawford MBE BSC (HONS) MB CHB FRCS (GLASG) FCEM
Chairman of the Board

British Red Cross
Dr. Vivien J. Armstrong MBBS DRCOG FRCA PGCE (FE)
Chief Medical Adviser

CONTRIBUTORS TO THE 5TH EDITION

Dr. Meng Aw-Yong BSC MBBS DFMS DFMB
Medical Adviser, St. John Ambulance
Jim Dorman
Operations Director, St. Andrew's First Aid
Joe Mulliga[...] of First Aid Education, British Red Cross

TRIPARTITE [...]IERCIAL COMMITTEE

St. John Am[...]e
Richard Eve[...]
Director of T[...] –
Richard Fern[...]
Head of Strat[...] ommunications
Andrew New[...]
Commercial Pr[...] Manager
St. Andrew's Fi[...] Aid
Helen Forrest
Head of Marketi[...]
Jim Dorman
Operations Direc[...]
British Red Cross
Anne McColl
Director of Education
Jude Holmes
Head of Education Marketing

AUTHORS' ACKNOWLEDGMENTS

The authors would like to extend special thanks to: the Clinical Directorate of St. John Ambulance; Stewart Simpson, Training Manager, St. Andrew's First Aid; Joslyn Kofi Opata, Administrator British Red Cross; Dr. Sarah Davidson, Head of Psychosocial Support, British Red Cross; Jane Keogh, Production Development Manager, First Aid Education, British Red Cross.

PUBLISHERS' ACKNOWLEDGMENTS

DK Publishing would like to thank: Sanjay Chauhan and Duncan Turner for design assistance; Daniel Stewart for organizing locations for photography; Sneha Sunder Benjamin for editorial assistance; Pallavi Singh and Vineetha Mokkil for proofreading; Sachin Gupta for technical assistance, and Bev Speight and Nigel Wright of XAB Design for art direction of the original photography shoots.
DK Publishing would also like to thank the following people who appear as models:
Lyndon Allen, Gillian Andrews, Kayko Andrieux, Mags Ashcroft, Nicholas Austin, Neil Bamfo[...] Jay Benedict, Dunstan Bentley, Joseph Bevan, Bob Bridle, Gerard Brown, Helen Brown, Jennifer Brown, Val Brown, Michelle Burke [...]lyn Calitz, Tyler Chambers, Evie Clark, Tim Clark, Junior Cole, Sue Cooper, Linda Dare, Julia Davies, Simon Davis, Tom Defrates, [...] Dick, Jemima Dunne, Maria Elia, Phil Fitzgerald, Alex Gayer, John Goldsmid, Nicholas Hayne, Stephen Hines, Nicola Hodgson [...]er Holbrook, Jennifer Irving, Dan James, Megan Jones, Dallas Kidman, Carol King, Ashwin Khurana, Andrea Kofi-Opata, Andrews [...]ata, Edna Kofi-Opata, Joslyn Kofi-Opata, Tim Lane, Libby Lawson, Wren Lawson-Foley, Daniel Lee, Crispin Lord, Danny Lo[...] iet Lord, Phil Lord, Gareth Lowe, Mulkina Mackay, Ethan Mackay-Wardle, Ben Marcus, Catherine McCormick, Fiona McDonald, Alfie McMeeking, Cath McMeeking, Archie Midgley, David Midgley, Eve Mills, Erica Mills, Gary Moore, Sandra Newman, Matt Robbins, Dean Morris, Eva Mulligan, Priscilla Nelson-Cole, Rachel NG, Emma Noppers, Phil Ormerod, Julie Oughton, Rebekah Parsons-King, Stefan Podohorodecki, Tom Raettig, Andrew Roff, Ian Rowland, Phil Sergeant, Vicky Short, Lucy Sims, Gregory Small, Andrew Smith, Emily Smith, Sophie Smith, Bev Speight, Silke Spingies, Michael Stanfield, Alex Stewart, Adam Stoneham, David Swinson, Hannah Swinson, Laura Swinson, Becky Tennant, Laura Tester, Pip Tinsley, Daniel Toorie, Helen Thewlis, Fiona Vance, Adam Walker, Jonathan Ward, David Wardle, Dion Wardle, Francesca Wardell, Angela Wilkes, Liz Wheeler, Jenny Woodcock, Nigel Wright, Nan Zhang.
Picture credits DK Publishing would like to thank the following for their kind permission to reproduce their photographs: Getty Images: Andrew Boyd 168–69.

All other images © Dorling Kindersley. For further information see www.dkimages.com